A FAREWELL TO VIROLOGY

A FAREWELL TO VIROLOGY

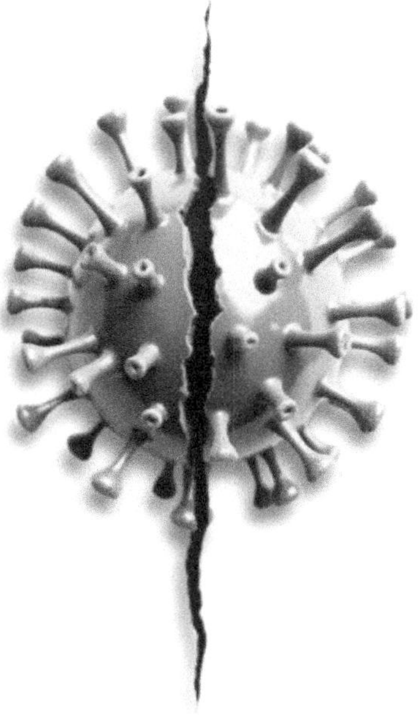

Dr Mark Bailey

A Farewell to Virology
First published by drsambailey.com in 2022
Print version first published in 2025
New Zealand

Paperback ISBN: 978-0-473-73667-5
Hardcover ISBN: 978-0-473-73668-2
PDF ISBN: 978-0-473-73670-5

CONTENTS

INTRODUCTION

By mid-2020, my wife Samantha and I thought that the "COVID" event would be over by Christmas. The narrative was so preposterous and was replete with so many contradictions that we believed the majority of people would reject the "countermeasures", including the vaccines in the pipeline. However, by early 2021 it was clearly apparent that the fraud was only growing. Most of the public was ensconced in the storyline and many continued to parrot the puerile marketing slogans aimed at mindlessly propagating and legitimising the "pandemic".

In November 2021, Dr John Bevan-Smith and I published *The COVID-19 Fraud & War on Humanity*.[1] The essay focussed on the pseudoscientific elements of "outbreak" modelling, the Polymerase Chain Reaction (PCR) in the creation of 'case' numbers, and "viral genomics". All of these elements had been employed to create the illusion of a "coronavirus" pandemic. However, the most important pillar of the fraud concerned 'isolation', that is, the very existence of the purported "virus":

> *Everything turns on these two concepts: absence and presence. Of what is SARS-CoV-2 predicated: absence or presence? That is the question we must decide. For without the instantiated presence of SARS-CoV-2 there are no COVID-19 cases to count, and therefore no ground or justification for any government's response to a phantom pandemic.*[2]

For many of us who could see this foundational aspect of the fraud, 2022 was the darkest year during the COVID-era. Many governments had successfully indoctrinated their citizenry into the acceptance of a two-

---

[1] Mark Bailey & John Bevan-Smith, "The COVID-19 Fraud & War on Humanity", 11 Nov 2021: https://drsambailey.com/covid-19/the-covid-19-fraud-war-on-humanity/

[2] Ibid.

tiered class system based on COVID vaccine passports. Furthermore, the "rules" could change on a monthly, if not weekly basis and countries took turns at brutally suppressing their populations. All of it was reliant on the fear-based narratives involving an alleged novel and dangerous "virus" (or one of its latest 'variants').

Unfortunately, many of the prominent individuals and organisations who were supposedly against the tyranny continued to uphold the foundational fraud: namely, the existence of SARS-CoV-2 as an infectious, disease-causing entity. Indeed, 2022 saw many of these "freedom" fighters ineptly start attacking those of us who had been exposing the pseudoscience of virology. As I wrote in the present essay:

> *In some cases these critics state that everything about the pandemic is a fraud,* except *the claim by the virologists (and the WHO) that SARS-CoV-2 has a physical existence as a pathogenic particle. They cannot see that the very basis of the fraud is also a fraud.* [Page 94]

One weakness for those of us taking the 'no virus' position was that there was no formal refutation of the entire virus model. There was the Perth Group's *HIV – a virus like no other,*[3] an uncontested 2017 treatise exposing the lack of evidence for "HIV" specifically. We also had the pivotal contributions from pioneers such as Dr Stefan Lanka and David Crowe. *Virus Mania*, first published in 2007 by Torsten Engelbrecht and Dr Claus Köhnlein was another instrumental publication that exposed virological fraud on a wider front including the media's role in propagating fear and promoting unnecessary pharmaceuticals.

In 2020 the COVID-19 fraud kindled a new wave of 'no virus' proponents such as Drs Andy Kaufman, Tom Cowan and Sam Bailey who rapidly took

---

[3] The Perth Group, "HIV - a virus like no other", 12 Jul 2017: http://theperthgroup.com/HIV/TPGVirusLikeNoOther.pdf

the information to millions of viewers. Every aspect of virological "science" was dissected in hundreds of video presentations and articles, building on the work of the aforementioned groundbreakers.

However, by 2022 I sensed an urgent need for a standalone treatise refuting the virus model. *A Farewell to Virology* was actually "repurposed" from another essay I was writing but was modified in the last month to take its final form.[4] It would have been ideal to have had more time to develop and refine the essay but there was an immediate feeling of relief when we published it on our website. The only mistakes that were found post-publication were in the form of some minor typographical errors.

Within a short time *A Farewell* had over 100,000 views and by 2024 it had over 250,000 views on our website alone. In 2023, film-maker Steve Falconer took on the difficult task of converting the text into a three-part video production and this also garnered hundreds of thousands of views across our platforms.[5] The essay has now been translated into multiple languages and has reached every corner of the world. Many people have written to us saying that it was this essay that definitively ended their belief in the existence of viruses. So even if it is a bit 'raw' in places, the message is certainly hitting its target.

A major theme throughout the essay is the lack of valid controls in the virologists' methodologies. Subsequent to the publication of *A Farewell* I realised there needed to be a formal outline explaining why their "gold standard" isolation technique *cannot* be controlled. Hence in 2024 I published *Virology's Event Horizon* which took the refutation of the virus model to the most foundational level. In essence, the cell culture method is nothing more than a smokescreen used by virologists to hide the

---

[4] See video description: https://drsambailey.com/resources/videos/viruses-unplugged/a-farewell-to-virology-part-three-dr-mark-bailey-and-steve-falconer/

[5] https://drsambailey.com/resources/videos/viruses-unplugged/a-farewell-to-virology-part-one/

deception that their "evidence" for viruses is based on assertion and not demonstration.

The critical factor is that "viruses" have never been discovered in nature and subsequently studied.*[6] As I have previously stated, virology invented itself as a pursuit before establishing whether or not the imagined entities actually existed.[7] That is why virology is a pseudoscience, and why its elaborate paraphernalia of cell cultures, electron microscopy, human and animal experiments, purported diagnostic tests and epidemiological data is nothing more than an elaborate subterfuge substituting presence for absence. Likewise, because none of the speculative premises on which virology is based have ever been established scientifically, we should not accept any new claims that are the product of more recent or new technology such as metagenomics or proteomics. Hence, *Virology's Event Horizon* has been included in this book to emphasise the importance of this fact.

Perhaps one oversight of *A Farewell* was not addressing bacteriophages and giant "viruses". These were included in *Virus, Bacteriophage & Single "Virus" Genomics*, an essay in which I also responded to "technological advancements" as purported evidence for the virus model:

> *While the notional virus model has changed over time, the underlying premise of a contagious disease-causing entity has never been established. Nevertheless, its proponents have attempted to incorporate naturally-observed particles such as "bacteriophages" into the virological realm without*

6 *Compare this to micro-organisms such as bacteria and fungi which can be found in nature and subsequently studied. See also footnote 225: There is no evidence that any micro-organisms *per se* have "pathogenic" abilities to invade healthy tissue and cause disease: https://drsambailey.com/resources/videos/germ-theory/why-pathogens-dont-exist/, however experiments with valid controls are possible with bacterial and fungal cells so the hypothesis can be tested.

7 Mark Bailey, "Warnings Signs You Have Been Tricked By Virologists...Again", 25 Jul 2022: https://drsambailey.com/warnings-signs-you-have-been-tricked-by-virologists-again/

> *establishing they are viruses, while portraying technological advances as the reason for their purported discovery.*[8]

In view of this potential oversight while endeavouring to expose the flaws in the virus model, the essay has also been included in this book. All of these essays, complete with their hyperlinks, can be freely downloaded at drsambailey.com.

[8] Mark Bailey, *Virus, Bacteriophage & Single "Virus" Genomics*, 20 Jul 2024: https://drsambailey.com/virus-bacteriophage-single-virus-genomics/

A FAREWELL TO VIROLOGY
(EXPERT EDITION)

ABSTRACT

Virology invented the virus model but has consistently failed to fulfil its own requirements. It is claimed that viruses cause disease after transmitting between hosts such as humans and yet the scientific evidence for these claims is missing. One of virology's greatest failures has been the inability to obtain any viral particles directly from the tissues of organisms said to have "viral" diseases. In order to obfuscate this state of affairs, virologists have resorted to creating their own pseudoscientific methods to replace the longstanding scientific method, as well as changing the dictionary meaning of words in order to support their anti-scientific practices. For instance, an "isolated" isolate does not require the physical existence of the particles in order to be afforded "isolation" status.

A viral particle must fulfil defined physical and biological properties including being a replication-competent intracellular parasite capable of *causing* disease in a host such as a human. However, "viruses" such as SARS-CoV-2 are nothing more than phantom constructs, existing only in imaginations and computer simulations. In this paradigm, cases of invented diseases like COVID-19 are nothing more than the detection of selected genetic sequences and proteins *purported* to be "viral." The existence of a virus is not required in this loop of circular reasoning and thus entire "pandemics" can be built upon digital creations and falsely sustained through *in vitro* ("test tube") molecular reactions.

This essay contains three parts. Part One outlines some of the history of virology and the failures of the virologists to follow the scientific method. The many and far-reaching claims of the virologists can all be shown to be flawed due to: (a) the lack of direct evidence, and (b) the invalidation of indirect "evidence" due to the uncontrolled nature of the experiments. The examples provided cover all major aspects of the virological fraud including alleged isolation, cytopathic effects, genomics, antibodies, and animal pathogenicity studies.

Part Two examines the fraud used to propagate the COVID-19 "pandemic." A breakdown of the methodology relied upon by the original inventors Fan Wu et al., shows how the fictional SARS-CoV-2 was "created" through anti-scientific methods and linguistic sleights of hands. It is part of an ongoing deception where viruses are claimed to exist by templating them against previous "virus" templates. Using SARS-CoV-2 as an example, the trail of "coronavirus" genomic templates going back to the 1980s reveals that none of these genetic sequences have ever been shown to come from inside any viral particle — the phylogenetic trees are fantasies. The misapplication of the polymerase chain reaction has propagated this aspect of virology's fraud and created the 'cases' to maintain the illusion of a pandemic.

Part Three provides an analysis of how some key participants, "health" institutions, and the mainstream media maintain the virus illusion through information control and narratives that parrot virology's claims. By way of happenstance, the virological fraud now finds itself front and centre of the COVID-19 fraud. From here, however, it can be critically appraised by those outside virology and the pseudo-scientific paradigm virology has built around itself can finally be dismantled and laid to rest.

The aim of this essay is to provide refutations to various claims that pathogenic viruses exist and cause disease. SARS-CoV-2 has been used as the main example but the principles apply to all alleged viruses. What follows addresses virology's often arcane literature on its own terms, which, it should be said, may make parts of this essay somewhat heavy reading. However, it is hoped that this contribution will fill a niche for the reader seeking a more technical understanding of the virus hypothesis as it seeks to expose the very foundation of purported pandemics and fraudulent medical practices. The threat of virology to humanity is increasing so it is time we bid farewell to these destructive pseudoscientific practices and free ourselves from unnecessary fears.

PART ONE

SARS-COV-2 NOT FOUND

Perhaps the primary evidence that the pathogenic viral theory is problematic is that no published scientific paper has ever shown that particles fulfilling the definition of viruses have been directly isolated and purified from any tissues or bodily fluids of any sick human or animal. Using the commonly accepted definition of "isolation", which is the separation of one thing from all other things, there is general agreement that this has never been done in the history of virology.

— Dr Thomas Cowan et al., The "Settling the Virus Debate Statement, 2022.[9]

As of 11 September 2022 and following extensive enquiries through Freedom of Information (FOI) requests coordinated by Christine Massey, not one of 209 mainly health or science institutions in over 35 countries have been able to provide direct evidence of the alleged SARS-CoV-2 virus.[10] The institutions were asked to produce any documents demonstrating, "the purification of 'SARS-CoV-2' said to have caused disease in humans (via maceration, filtration, and use of an ultracentrifuge; also referred to at times by some people as 'isolation'), directly from a diseased human..." On many occasions, following an admission that no such evidence is held, institutions such as the New Zealand Ministry of Health then suggest that, "there are several examples

---

[9] Thomas Cowan, et al., "The 'Settling the Virus Debate' Statement", 14 Jul 2022: https://drsambailey.com/resources/settling-the-virus-debate/

[10] Christine Massey, "209 health/science institutions globally all failed to cite even 1 record of 'SARS-COV-2' purification, by anyone, anywhere, ever": https://www.fluoridefreepeel.ca/68-health-science-institutions-globally-all-failed-to-cite-even-1-record-of-sars-cov-2-purification-by-anyone-anywhere-ever/ (accessed 11 Sep 2022.)

of the virus being isolated and cultured in a laboratory setting."[11] However, the examples referred to are universally tissue culture proxy experiments, in which the word 'isolation' has become detached from its understood meaning and it has not been demonstrated that any particle, imaged or imagined, has the properties of a disease-causing virus. In any case, it is a distraction from the wider issue exposed by the FOI requests, which is that particles claimed to be viruses can never be found in human subjects. Virology has made excuses for this missing evidence but even allowing for this embarrassing deficiency, it is running out of places to hide as its various methodologies are increasingly scrutinised by those outside the field. This essay outlines the many aspects of virology's anti-science that have been employed to maintain the illusion that pathogenic viruses exist. The situation has become increasingly dangerous and since early 2020, the COVID-19 "pandemic" has been used as a Trojan horse to bring humanity to its knees.

DR SIOUXSIE WILES — VIROLOGY'S 'ISOLATION' ACOLYTE

> *The density gradient centrifugation is the scientifically required standard technique for the demonstration of the existence of a virus. Despite the fact that this method is described in all microbiology manuals as the "virus isolation technique", it is never applied in experiments meant to demonstrate the existence of pathogenic viruses.*
>
> — Dr Stefan Lanka, 2015.[12]

The defence of virology's methodologies is obviously attempted by its promoters, including New Zealand government and state-funded media's

---

[11] NZ Ministry of Health, "Official Information Act response Ref: H202102878": https://drive.google.com/drive/folders/1okJiB4PdWN3tiei_g67zTUfok92kuqqS

[12] Stefan Lanka, "The Virus Misconception", *WISSEnSCHAFFTPLUS magazin*, 06/2015: https://www.researchgate.net/publication/316280466_Virology_State_of_the_Art

favoured microbiologist Siouxsie Wiles.[13] Her employer, the University of Auckland, is among those institutions who have now confirmed that, "[it] has not done any work relating to the purification of any Covid-19 virus,"[14] and therefore has neither found in, nor isolated from, any human subject the so-called virus named SARS-CoV-2. This associate professor, who advised the country that, "the world is on fire," in March 2020,[15] was ordained New Zealander of the Year in 2021 for, "helping millions globally see past the fear and complexities of the pandemic...and helping to keep us safe."[16] In her November 2020 article, "Koch's postulates, COVID, and misinformation rabbit holes," Wiles alleged that, "the people asking for evidence of the existence of the SARS-CoV-2 virus responsible for COVID-19 are specifically wording their request to rule out obtaining any evidence that the virus exists."[17] Her article quickly went off on a tangent about Koch's Postulates being unsuitable for viruses and she thus declared them as invalid in that context. It is unclear why she did not mention Rivers Postulates,[18] which were designed specifically to include viruses, although perhaps because she would have to admit that these postulates have never been fulfilled either. And while Koch's Postulates relate to the

---

13 https://unidirectory.auckland.ac.nz/profile/s-wiles

14 Christine Massey, https://www.fluoridefreepeel.ca/fois-reveal-that-health-science-institutions-around-the-world-have-no-record-of-sars-cov-2-isolation-purification/

15 "Microbiologist Siouxsie Wiles gives advice on preventing coronavirus", *1News*, 16 Mar 2020: https://www.youtube.com/watch?v=u_YVN7KYzhA&t=43s

16 Nikki Preston, "Passionate microbiologist Siouxsie Wiles named as New Zealander of the Year", *NZ Herald*, 1 Apr 2021: https://www.nzherald.co.nz/nz/passionate-microbiologist-siouxsie-wiles-named-as-new-zealander-of-the-year; "Dr Siouxsie Wiles MNZM", New Zealander of the Year Awards (undated, accessed 22 May 21), 2: https://nzawards.org.nz/winners/dr-siouxsie-wiles-mnzm/. The citation for the award reads as follows: "In the face of considerable criticism – on her authority, on her appearance, on her gender – Siouxsie's continued to respond to one of the greatest challenges of our time with empathy, innovation and courage, and her work has been seen by millions and even used by governments and organisations as part of their official pandemic communications."

17 Siouxsie Wiles, "Koch's postulates, Covid, and misinformation rabbit holes", 16 Nov 2020: https://www.auckland.ac.nz/en/news/2020/11/16/kochs-postulates-covid-and-misinformation-rabbit-holes.html

18 Thomas Rivers, "Viruses and Koch's Postulates", *Journal of Bacteriology*, 33/1, 1937.

establishment of disease-causation and contagion, rather than the specific issue of whether viral particles can be found in or from human subjects, she could have simply explained that the virologists have spent much of the 20th century trying to identify viruses directly from sick humans without any success. Wiles then fallaciously introduced Falkow's Molecular Postulates[19] into her argument, providing no explanation as to how they could be employed to demonstrate the physical existence of the claimed SARS-CoV-2 in a human or anywhere else.

Awkwardly for Wiles, the World Health Organization (WHO) stated in 2003 that with regard to SARS-CoV-1, "conclusive identification of a causative [agent] must meet all criteria in the so-called 'Koch's Postulate [*sic*].' The additional experiments needed to fulfil these criteria are currently under way at a laboratory in the Netherlands."[20] The WHO's article was removed from its website without explanation in 2021 but is still able to be accessed through the Internet Archive.[21] The fanciful claim that Koch's Postulates were met in 2003 by Fouchier et al. with SARS-CoV-1 has been refuted elsewhere.[22] Their monkey experiment was not only invalidated by its lack of controls and unnatural exposure route but like all virology publications, they failed to demonstrate a particle that met the definition of a virus. Wiles also appeared to be at odds with Na Zhu et al., one of the first teams that claimed to have discovered SARS-CoV-2, because they

---

19 Falkow's Molecular Postulates: "(1) The phenotype or property under investigation should be associated with pathogenic members of a genus or pathogenic strains of a species. (2) Specific inactivation of the gene(s) associated with the suspected virulence trait should lead to a measurable loss in pathogenicity or virulence. (3) Reversion or allelic replacement of the mutated gene should lead to restoration of pathogenicity." - Stanley Falkow, "Molecular Koch's Postulates Applied to Microbial Pathogenicity", *Reviews of Infectious Diseases*, Jul-Aug 1988: https://pubmed.ncbi.nlm.nih.gov/3055197/

20 WHO, "Severe Acute Respiratory Syndrome (SARS) - multi-country outbreak - Update 12", 27 Mar 2003.

21 https://web.archive.org/web/20030802232208/http://www.who.int/csr/don/2003_03_27b/en/

22 Torsten Engelbrecht, et al., *Virus Mania*, 3rd English Edition, Books on Demand, 2021, 2: Samantha Bailey, "What Happened To SARS-1?", 27 Jan 2021: https://drsambailey.com/resources/videos/viruses-unplugged/what-happened-to-sars-1/

conceded that, "although our study does not fulfill Koch's postulates, our analyses provide evidence implicating 2019-nCoV [later 'SARS-CoV-2'] in the Wuhan outbreak. Additional evidence to confirm the etiologic significance of 2019-nCoV in the Wuhan outbreak include...animal (monkey) experiments to provide evidence of pathogenicity."[23]

> — *However, whether different virologists want to entertain the validity of Koch's Postulates or not, it is simply another distraction as* ***the postulates require the physical isolation of a microbe*** *rather than assertions that one exists through means such as computer simulations, imaging vesicles of unknown biological function, or claiming that unpurified biological soups given to animals contain "viruses".*

Wiles also decided to champion virology's blatant misuse of the word 'isolation' when she stated, "as for using isolation in the every-day sense of the word, rather than the definition that is relevant to the question being asked? Well, that's just bloody ridiculous and a clear sign these requests for evidence are not being made in good faith."[24] She appeared to be incredulous that others had pointed out that the definition of a word being used scientifically was unilaterally changed by the virologists to imply a certain proof was obtained. However, if their use of isolation does not mean what most people think it means, then it is likely that most of the public are being misinformed. On this account, Wiles is an active participant in promulgating disinformation, whether it is an act of wilful blindness or otherwise. Wiles needs to show her hand as an expert and explain to the public what the definition of isolation in virology means, in particular with regard to demonstrating the putative existence of viruses.

---

[23] Na Zhu et al., "A Novel Coronavirus from Patients with Pneumonia in China, 2019", The *New England Journal of Medicine*, 382 (20 Feb 2020, first published 24 Jan 2020, updated 29 Jan 2020), 728: https://pubmed.ncbi.nlm.nih.gov/31978945/

[24] Siouxsie Wiles, "Koch's postulates, Covid, and misinformation rabbit holes", 16 Nov 2020: https://www.auckland.ac.nz/en/news/2020/11/16/kochs-postulates-covid-and-misinformation-rabbit-holes.html

Perhaps she thinks she did explain when she wrote, "when virologists want to isolate a virus from a sample they'll take the sample or some part of it and add it to some cells – usually ones that are relatively easy to grow in the lab – and then look to see if the cells die and/or if there are any virus particles released into the liquid nutrient bath the cells are growing in."[25] It is unclear if Wiles is implying that the "virus isolate" is established by: (a) the taking of the sample, (b) seeing some cells die *in vitro*, (c) the release of claimed "virus particles" in the tissue culture, or (d) all or some combination of these elements. However, nothing she described requires the existence of viruses — it is a game of deception, whether realised or not. It simply involves the assertion that a virus was in the sample, blaming the breakdown of experimentally stressed cells in the test tube on the imagined virus, and then declaring that some of the vesicles (whose biological composition and function were not established) were the viruses. There is a further fatal flaw in this exercise. As this essay will detail, the claims that SARS-CoV-2 has been shown to exist through this methodology are all scientifically invalid as *none* of the experiments were performed with valid controls.

This is exemplary of how Wiles has acted in her role as one of the key influencers for the New Zealand government's disinformation campaign and its murderous rollout programme of an injectable product called Comirnaty™ – claiming that non-specific tissue culture experiments verify the existence of the virus when nothing of the kind has been demonstrated. The issue extends beyond just SARS-CoV-2 — *every* virus asserted to exist relies on similar pseudoscience. The history of virology reveals that the types of cells eventually selected for these experiments have been those that have a propensity to breakdown with the claim of virus-induced 'cytopathic effects' (CPEs), rather than those that are, "relatively easy to grow in the lab," as Wiles claimed in her article. For

[25] Ibid.

example, Vero E6 monkey cells[26] have long been favoured by virologists, supposedly due to their "suitability" to host many viruses, but suspiciously also, because the aneuploid[27] kidney line is more susceptible to toxic insults from additional ingredients such as the ubiquitous nephrotoxic antibiotics and antifungals added to the culture mix. When one group attempted to culture SARS-CoV-2, they had no desired result with human adenocarcinoma cells (A549), human liver cells (HUH7.0), human embryonic kidney cells (HEK-293T), and a big brown bat kidney cell line (EFK3B), but then declared they had a "viral isolate" following the observation of CPEs in Vero E6 cells.[28] As is typical, there seemed to be no sense of irony for them that the purported human respiratory virus cannot be shown to "infect" the relevant cell type, let alone the relevant species. And their experiments were once again invalidated by the absence of appropriate control cultures.

WHY ISOLATION MATTERS

He who controls the language controls the masses.

— Saul Alinsky[29]

A further embarrassment for virology is that alleged viral particles that have been successfully purified have not been shown to be replication-competent or disease-causing by themselves. In other words, what have been physically isolated can only be said to be extracellular vesicles (EVs). In May 2020, a publication appeared in the journal *Viruses* that claimed, "nowadays, it is an almost impossible mission to separate EVs and viruses

---

[26] ATCC, "VERO C1008 [Vero 76, clone E6, Vero E6]": https://www.atcc.org/products/crl-1586

[27] Aneuploidy means the presence of an abnormal number of chromosomes in a cell.

[28] Jennifer Harcourt, et al., "Severe Acute Respiratory Syndrome Coronavirus 2 from Patient with Coronavirus Disease, United States", *Emerging Infectious Diseases*, June 2020: https://wwwnc.cdc.gov/eid/article/26/6/20-0516_article

[29] *Rules for Radicals*, Random House, 1971.

by means of canonical vesicle isolation methods, such as differential ultracentrifugation, because they are frequently co-pelleted due to their similar dimension."[30] 'Nowadays' means in contrast to the past and it is unclear how such an observed technical change may be reconciled with biological laws. It appears more likely that the virologists are distancing themselves from their own techniques in order to avoid refutation of their own postulates. They may have to accept that the reason differential ultracentrifugation is not able to separate viruses from other vesicles is because their assertion that viruses are present in the sample is ill-founded.

The virologists are clearly distracting from the foundational issue of isolation as they have been unable to deliver on this front. Instead of addressing the problem honestly and scientifically, they have obfuscated the language. In 2017, The Perth Group pointed out in their *magnum opus,* "HIV - a virus like no other" that, "in virology, while purification retains its everyday meaning, 'isolation' is an expediential term virologists assign to data they claim are proof a particular virus exists."[31] In other words, it is convenient and practical but with regard to the claims that are made and the subsequent actions that are carried out against humanity, it should be viewed as improper and immoral. In the same essay, The Perth Group documented the following examples of virologists adapting the scientific language, as suited, for their own purposes:

> *HIV expert Jay Levy defines virus isolation as a "sample of a virus from a defined source", White and Fenner as the ability to "identify a totally unforeseen virus, or even discover an entirely new agent". Montagnier and Weiss as "propagating them [viruses] in cells in culture". The 2013 sixth edition of*

[30] Flavia Giannessi, et al., "The Role of Extracellular Vesicles as Allies of HIV, HCV and SARS Viruses", *Viruses,* 22 May 2020: https://www.ncbi.nlm.nih.gov/pmc/articles/PMC7291340/

[31] The Perth Group, "HIV - a virus like no other", 12 Jul 2017: http://theperthgroup.com/HIV/TPGVirusLikeNoOther.pdf

> *Fields Virology defines isolation as "Viruses can be isolated from an infected host by harvesting excreted or secreted material, blood, or tissue and testing for induction of the original symptoms in the identical host, or induction of some abnormal pathology in a substitute host, or in a cell culture...Once the presence of a virus has been established, it is often desirable to prepare a genetically pure clone". It goes without saying that if virus isolation is to "take a sample of a virus from a defined source", or "propagating them in cells in culture", one first must have proof the virus exists in "a defined source" or "in cells in culture". Neither is virus isolation "induction of some abnormal pathology" or "once the presence of a virus has been established".*[32]

It is a travesty that this state of affairs exists and the grossly misleading practice renders virology's many claims of isolation as unsubstantiated. But do the virologists themselves offer any explanation for their relentless abuse of the English language? In 2021, veteran virologist Professor Vincent Racaniello explained, even with regard to the definition of fundamental terms such as 'isolate' that, "what happens is you're trained in someone's laboratory and you hear them say things and you associate a meaning with them and that's what you do, and they may or may not be right."[33] In the same presentation, Racaniello himself didn't appear to notice a problem with his own definition of what are supposed to be scientific terms when he went on to say, "an isolate is a virus that we have isolated from an infected host and we have propagated that in culture." Ironically, in a 2015 article, regarding appropriate scientific terminology and the word 'transfection',[34] Racaniello stated, "if you view the English

---

[32] Ibid.

[33] Vincent Racaniello, "Virus isolates, variants, strains - what are they?", *Vincent Racaniello*, 2 Mar 2021: https://www.youtube.com/watch?v=G2G2bWUAef0&t=75s

[34] "Transfection is a process of introducing nucleic acid into eukaryotic cells using various chemical or physical methods", from *Comprehensive Biotechnology*, 2nd edition, Elsevier, 2011.

language as a dynamic means of communication that continually evolves and provides words with new meanings, then this incorrect use of transfection probably does not bother you. But scientists must be precise in their use of language, otherwise their ability to communicate will be impaired."[35] An analysis of Racaniello's presentation on viral isolation and the misuse of language in science has been dealt with previously by Dr Samantha Bailey in, "The Truth About Virus Isolation."[36] It is illustrative of the problem where multiple generations of virologists appear trapped in a world of semantic circular reasoning, albeit with differing degrees of insight.

Virology invented the hypothesis of viruses so whatever method it employs in an attempt to prove their existence, it must satisfy that definition. At the heart of the matter is a simple concept and we need to see evidence that alleged disease-causing particles cause new particles that are clones of the former. Claiming that detected proteins and nucleic acids are of a specific viral origin is not possible unless the alleged viral particles have been truly isolated by purification and shown to have these key biological characteristics. As outlined by The Perth Group in, "HIV - a virus like no other," purification is necessary to prove the existence of viruses for several reasons, including the following:

1. *Viruses replicate only in living cells. Since cells and viruses are composed of the same biochemical constituents, separation of particles from cellular material is essential for defining which nucleic acid and proteins belong to the virus particles.*
2. *To prove the particles are infectious. In other words, it is particles, not other factors, that are responsible for the*

---

35 Vincent Racaniello, "What does transfection mean?", *Virology blog*, 12 Feb 2015: https://www.virology.ws/2015/02/12/what-does-transfection-mean/

36 Samantha Bailey, "The Truth About Virus Isolation", 14 Apr 2021: https://drsambailey.com/resources/videos/viruses-unplugged/the-truth-about-virus-isolation/

production of new particles. This requires purification of both sets of particles.

3. *To demonstrate their biological and pathological effects.*
4. *To obtain antigens (proteins) and nucleic acids for use in antibody and genomic tests respectively.*[37]

Although less common, virologists will sometimes obfuscate the meaning of 'purification' as well. On 23 May 2022, Belgian Professor of Virology Marc Van Ranst[38] claimed that with regard to SARS-CoV-2, "in another article (https://europepmc.org/article/pmc/pmc7122600) they have further purified the virus by ultracentrifugation in beta-cyclodextrin."[39] Van Ranst was referring to a 2008 paper that described, "large-Scale preparation of UV-Inactivated SARS coronavirus virions," which related to the purported SARS-CoV-1 virus.[40] However, this paper simply outlines a protocol *claiming* to purify virions and there is no part of the paper that demonstrated the existence of any replication-competent particle — all that was shown were some low quality images purporting to show "infected" Vero E6 cells. (See next section regarding 'cytopathic effects'.) With regard to the "check of purified virions" following centrifugation, no images were provided but the claim was made that, "the concentration of purified virions is determined by BCA [bicinchoninic acid] assay with BSA [bovine serum albumin] as a standard." This was an unfounded conclusion as the BCA assay simply measures the total concentration of protein in a solution — the technique is unable to provide evidence that there are any "virions" present in a sample.

---

37 The Perth Group, "HIV - a virus like no other", 12 Jul 2017: http://theperthgroup.com/HIV/TPGVirusLikeNoOther.pdf

38 "Marc Van Ranst", Wikispooks: https://wikispooks.com/wiki/Marc_Van_Ranst

39 By email from Marc Van Ranst, "Purification of SARS-CoV-2", 23 May 2022: https://www.fluoridefreepeel.ca/wp-content/uploads/2022/06/Belgium-Marc-Van-Ranst-May-2022-PACKAGE.pdf

40 Yasuko Tsunetsugu-Yokota, "Large-scale preparation of UV-inactivated SARS coronavirus virions for vaccine antigen", *Methods in Molecular Biology*, 1 Jan 2008: https://doi.org/10.1007/978-1-59745-181-9_11

Figure 1 below is an image purporting to show purified "bat SARS-like coronavirus" virions and was published in *Nature* in 2013 — the caption explains why such a declaration is ludicrous. (The convenient variation in particle size is apparently because, "[coronaviruses] usually have a diameter, excluding projections, of between 80 and 120 nm, although in extreme cases the diameter can vary between 60 and 220 nm."[41])

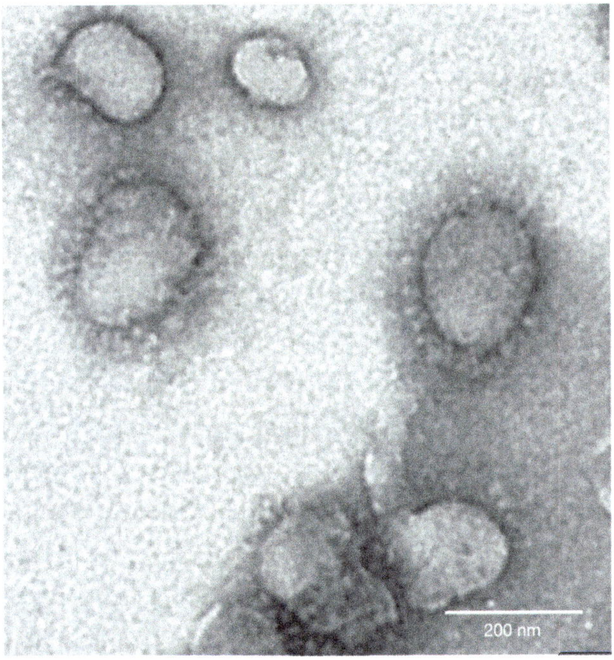

Figure 1. This image was described as, "[an] electron micrograph of purified virions," obtained by, "ultracentrifugation through a 20% sucrose cushion (5 ml) at 80,000g for 90 min using a Ty90 rotor (Beckman)." Aside from the fact that the biological properties of these imaged vesicles were not established, there is no indication that anything in the Vero E6 cell culture has been purified and no other contextual images were provided. Additionally, no control culture micrographs were documented. Source: Xing-Yi Ge, et al., "Isolation and characterization of a bat SARS-like coronavirus that uses the ACE2 receptor," *Nature*, 30 Oct 2013: https://doi.org/10.1038/nature12711 (See also page 81 with regard to the claim that Ralph Baric et al. utilised these "viruses" to create new ones.)

[41] Malcom MacNaughton and Heather Davies, "Coronaviridae", in *Animal Virus Structure*, Elsevier, 1987.

Likewise, the claim in Van Ranst's cited paper that, "it is better to confirm the amount of virion by 10% SDS-PAGE,"[42] is just as erroneous as this is simply a gel electrophoresis process to separate out proteins by their molecular mass — it cannot provide evidence that the proteins belong to a virus. Van Ranst also stated, "we can already detect the viral RNA in clinical samples. We can complete the viral genome decipher. We can grow the virus in cell culture and inoculate it into animal models and induce disease."[43] It is unknown whether Van Ranst appreciated that the uncontrolled methodologies being employed in all such experiments do not provide the required evidence for any "virus." So, when Van Ranst made the claim that, "no scientist doubts the existence of SARS-CoV-2,"[44] it makes one wonder whether the virologists will now have to change the definition of 'scientist' to maintain the delusive practices?

Van Ranst was not the only virologist making claims about purifying viruses though. In response to an email enquiry, Dr Marica Grossegesse[45] from the Robert Koch Institute responded that, "we purified SARS particles by density gradient. However, just from the cell culture derived virus, as you wrote. The challenge with purifying SARS from patient samples is that you won't get a visible band."[46] Apart from the imprecise terminology in substituting the name of a syndrome ('SARS' is severe acute respiratory syndrome) for a postulated virus, no further evidence was supplied as to how these claims were established. Presumably, Grossegesse is also using the definitions of "purification" and "virus" as depicted in Figure 1? In any case, when pressed for further details about

---

[42] Sodium Dodecyl Sulfate-PolyAcrylamide Gel Electrophoresis

[43] By email from Marc Van Ranst, "Purification of SARS-CoV-2", 23 May 2022: https://www.fluoridefreepeel.ca/wp-content/uploads/2022/06/Belgium-Marc-Van-Ranst-May-2022-PACKAGE.pdf

[44] Ibid.

[45] https://www.researchgate.net/profile/Marica-Grossegesse

[46] By email from Marica Grossegesse, Robert Koch Institute, "SARS-CoV-2 / questions", 1 Apr 2022: https://www.fluoridefreepeel.ca/wp-content/uploads/2022/07/RKI-Marcia-Grossegesse-controls-PACKAGE-redacted.pdf

how the experiments were controlled she responded, "we are not allowed to share any protocols with a private person. I can only refer to our publications, where infection experiments are described in detail." It appears that 'detail' has taken on a different meaning as well, as the publications failed to disclose the straightforward answers concerning controls being sought.

The area of isolation is one of the domains where virology is completely unhinged and as this essay will outline, SARS-CoV-2 remains nothing more than a hypothetical computer construct, assembled from genetic fragments of unproven provenance. There has never been a physically isolated (i.e. purified) particle shown to be responsible for the production of identical particles or a particle shown to be the cause of pathological effects in any human or in an experimental animal model. Thus, the declaration by virologists such as Van Ranst, along with the WHO and its adherents, that an infectious particle termed 'SARS-CoV-2' is causing a disease pandemic is shown to be patent scientific and intellectual fraud.

WHAT IS VIROLOGY?

> *When startled, the bird will take off and fly around in ever-decreasing circles until it manages to fly up its own backside, disappearing completely, which adds to its rarity.*
>
> — The mythical 'oozlum bird'.[47]

It is hard to know exactly what to call virology, but it is not science. The current practitioners are engaging in some form of algorithmic or statistical speculation added to circular reasoning and confirmation bias, with a complete absence of what should be the corresponding process of refutation that lies at the heart of the scientific method. While the abandonment of the scientific method may be unnoticed or accidental by

[47] Bill Wannan, *Crooked Mick of the Speewah: And Other Tall Tales*, Lansdowne, 1966.

lower level participants, there are almost certainly conspiratorial motivations at higher levels of the global hierarchy. For example, the WHO, the Centers for Disease Control (CDC) and the United Kingdom's Health Security Agency are all parties to virology's deceptive practices, as will be exposed in this essay. However, the anti-scientific practices are replicated in most other countries, whether this relates to claims of virus isolation and the wholesale misapplication of the polymerase chain reaction (PCR) for clinical diagnostics,[48] or a failure to disclose the crucial control details involved in virus culture and genome creation, which is the focus of much of this essay.

How is it that we test a scientific theory? Karl Popper expressed the centrality of refutation of a theory or hypothesis, thus:

> *So it is, I hold, the possibility of overthrowing it, or its falsifiability, that constitutes the possibility of testing it, and therefore the scientific character of a theory; and the fact that all tests of a theory are attempted falsifications of predictions derived with its help, furnishes the clue to the scientific method. This view of the scientific method is corroborated by the history of science, which shows that scientific theories are often overthrown by experiments, and that the overthrow of theories is indeed the vehicle of scientific process. The contention that science is circular cannot be upheld.*[49]

It is thus a reasonable question to ask has virology ever been a scientific pursuit? With regard to the scientific method, the virologists create

---

[48] Mark Bailey & John Bevan-Smith, "The COVID-19 Fraud & War on Humanity", 11 Nov 2021: https://drsambailey.com/covid-19/the-covid-19-fraud-war-on-humanity/

[49] Karl Popper, *The Open Society and its Enemies: Volume II The High Tide of Prophecy: Hegel, Marx, and the Aftermath* (London: Routledge & Kegan Paul (1962, first published 1947), 260.

unfalsifiable hypotheses by setting up paradigms where any number of observations, whether it be illness or alleged test results can be attributed to their 'viruses'. The observations are passed off as proof of virus existence in the manner of a circular loop of reasoning that no longer requires the demonstrable existence of a virus. Any claims of reproducibility, for example, in the form of a PCR process or a purported viral genome, are simply more circuits of the same loop.

Historically, virology has been characterised by a lack of valid control experiments and none of its foundational claims have been established through proper exercise of the scientific method. The first alleged virus to be discovered was the Tobacco Mosaic Virus and one of the proofs for this is said to be contained in Dmitri Ivanovsky's 1903 treatise *Über die Mosaikkrankheit der Tabakspflanze (About the Mosaic Disease of the Tobacco Plant).*[50] However, it is patently clear that Ivanovsky's described experiments lacked any valid control comparisons and were thus unscientific and inconclusive. He even commented that, "this disease finds favourable conditions of existence only in coastal regions. Such a conclusion fully agrees with the above observations concerning the influence of moisture on the development of the disease. Mosaic disease appears to be unique to humid and warm climates."[51] However, as germ theory was developing into the predominant disease-causation ideology at that time, rather than concluding that the Mosaic Disease was caused by environmental conditions, Ivanovsky concluded he had discovered an invisible virus.

It is perhaps tempting to forgive the early pioneers that their uncontrolled and unscientific methodologies were simply typical practices for that era. However, germ theory critic Claude Bernard offered the following insight into the importance of controls when adhering to the scientific method decades earlier in 1865: "If indeed we characterise experiment by a

---

[50] Dmitri Ivanovsky, "Über die Mosaikkrankheit der Tabakspflanze", *Zeitschrift für Pflanzenkrankheiten,* Vol. 13, No. 1, 1903, 1-41.

[51] Ibid.

variation or disturbance brought into a phenomenon, it is only in so far as we imply that the disturbance must be compared with the normal state. As experiments indeed are only judgments, they necessarily require comparison between two things; and the intentional or active element in an experiment is really the comparison which the mind intends to make."[52] Bernard was advising the need to have a valid control, or some suitable comparison to ensure it was only the new experimental element that was causing an outcome. Thus, the most charitable we could be is to suggest that perhaps some of the early virus hunters were unaware of the importance of the scientific method in their enthusiastic and unbridled pursuit of invisible enemies.

Moving forward to another early claimed virus discovery, the textbook *Retroviruses* informs us that, "in 1911, Peyton Rous at the Rockefeller Institute in New York reported the cell-free transmission of a sarcoma in chickens...The virus isolated by Rous bears the name of its discoverer: Rous sarcoma virus."[53] However a review of Rous' paper, "A Sarcoma of the Fowl,"[54] reveals that he did not claim to isolate anything, let alone anything that met the definition of a virus. His methodology involved grinding up chicken tumour material, filtering it, and injecting it directly into other chickens with the observation that some of them would also develop tumours. He reported that the "control" experiments consisted of injecting *unfiltered* tumour material into chickens which tended to result in much larger tumours. Rous postulated the presence of a causative ultramicroscopic organism but conceded that, "an agency of another sort is not out of the question." Indeed, the experiment failed to provide any evidence of an infectious and replicating particle. It simply showed that diseased tissue introduced by an unnatural and invasive route into another animal could cause it to exhibit a similar disease process.

---

[52] Claude Bernard, *An Introduction to the Study of Experimental Medicine,* 1865, translated by Henry Greene, Schuman Inc., 1949.

[53] *Retroviruses*, Cold Spring Harbor Laboratory Press, New York, 1997.

[54] Peyton Rous, "A Sarcoma of the Fowl Transmissible by an Agent Separable from the Tumor Cells", *J Exp Med*, 1 Apr 2022: https://doi.org/10.1084/jem.13.4.397

The claim that in 1925 pathologist William Gye demonstrated Rous had found a virus is also false. He merely asserted that a virus was at work in these experiments and conspicuously stated, "I wish particularly to stress one aspect of the search for the invisible viruses, and that is that the animal test is the final proof of the presence of the organism in an inoculum."[55] Again, the "final proof" did not involve the actual identification of an infectious organism in the inoculum — it simply demonstrated tumour formation following injection of diseased tissue. Further, it was determined in 1927 that sarcoma of the fowl could be induced by the injection of dilute arsenious acid and foreign embryonic pulp.[56] The carcinogenic effects were also replicated following the equivalent bacteriological filtration that Rous performed and the disease was shown to arise from the foreign tissue, not from the host tissues. The viral hypothesis should have been thrown out but half a century later the establishment kept it alive and rewarded Rous with a Nobel prize in 1966 for, "his discovery of tumour-inducing viruses."[57]

In 1954, when John Enders and Thomas Peebles claimed they had propagated the measles virus in human and monkey kidneys cells,[58] no further tolerance should have been extended to virology's unscientific experiments. Enders and Peebles added throat washings and blood to their cell cultures and on observing CPEs, or dying and breaking down cells in their test tubes, concluded that the *in vitro* appearances, "might be associated with the virus of measles." They did warn that, "cytopathic

---

[55] William Gye, "Discussion on Filter-Passing Viruses and Cancer", *BMJ*, 1 Aug 1925: https://www.jstor.org/stable/25445900

[56] A. W. M. White, "A Study of Sarcoma of the Fowl Produced by Arsenic and Embryonic Pulp", *The Journal of Cancer Research*, 1 Mar 1927: https://aacrjournals.org/jcancerres/article/11/1/111/449689/A-Study-of-Sarcoma-of-the-Fowl-Produced-by-Arsenic

[57] "The Nobel Prize in Physiology or Medicine 1966": https://www.nobelprize.org/prizes/medicine/1966/summary/

[58] John Enders and William Peebles, "Propagation in Tissue Cultures of Cytopathogenic Agents from Patients with Measles", *Proceedings of the Society for Experimental Biology and Medicine (PSEBM)*, 86 (received 16 May 1954), 277-286.

effects which superficially resemble those resulting from infection by the measles agents may possibly be induced by other viral agents present in the monkey kidney tissue or by unknown factors," but went on to inappropriately conclude that, "this group of agents is composed of representatives of the viral species responsible for measles."[59] Enders and Peebles performed no control experiments to check whether the culture procedure itself, that is the stressing of the cells in a test tube, would produce the same CPEs, thereby invalidating the evidence for their conclusion. Ideally, several control experiments should have been done: some with no human-derived samples added, some with human-derived samples from well subjects, and some with human-derived samples from unwell subjects, but said not to have measles clinically or some other alleged "viral" condition.

The virologists however, have continued to repeat the uncontrolled methodology of Enders and to this day claim that such CPEs are incontestable evidence of viruses. Dr Stefan Lanka has documented the history of these unscientific practices,[60] and in 2021 demonstrated that CPEs could be induced in cell cultures by the laboratory process itself.[61] The results of Lanka's experiments are depicted in Figure 2. In many virology publications a control or 'mock-infected' experiment is mentioned but the details of such experiments are conspicuous by their absence. A Northwestern University, Illinois webpage states that mock-infected means, "a control used in infection experiments. Two specimens are used, one that is infected with the virus/vector of interest and the other is treated the same way except without the virus."[62] The definition is already problematic as terms such as 'virus' and 'infected' have been introduced

---

59 Ibid.

60 Stefan Lanka, "The Virus Misconception", *WISSEnSCHAFFTPLUS magazin*, 01/2020, 4.

61 Dean Braus, "CPE - Control Experiment - 21 April 2021 - English version": https://odysee.com/@DeansDanes:1/cpe-english:f

62 Northwestern University, Illinois, "mock-infected" definition: https://groups.molbiosci.northwestern.edu/holmgren/Glossary/Definitions/Def-M/mock-infected.html

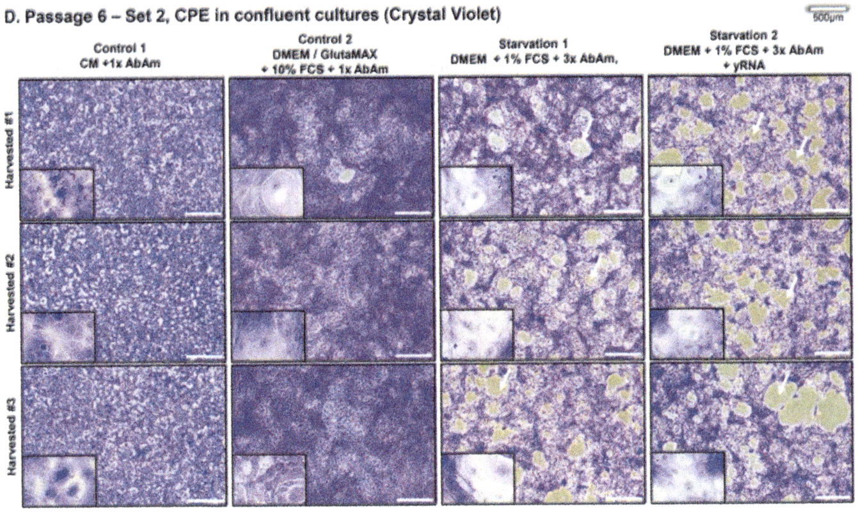

Figure 2. Dr Stefan Lanka's experiments: CPEs (white arrows) were induced by stressing the epithelial cells with passaging and antibiotics. The addition of yeast RNA (4th column) induced even more CPEs. No "viruses" were added and the experiments were performed in triplicate. Source: Stefan Lanka, et al., "Präliminäre Resultate der Kontrollversuche – Die Reaktion primärer humaner Epithelzellen auf stringente Virusamplifikations-Bedingungen widerlegen die Existenzbehauptungen aller Viren und von SARS-CoV-2", 25 Mar 2022: https://coldwelliantimes.com/eilmeldung/kontrollexperiment

and thus presumed to exist before being established. In any case, as will become clear, those involved in alleged virus isolation and genome creation are certainly not treating the mock-infected specimen in the same way minus the 'virus', and can be disingenuous or blatantly obstructive when pressed to admit this fact.

In June 2022, in response to an Official Information Act (OIA) request concerning the paper, "Characterization of the First SARS-CoV-2 Isolates from Aotearoa New Zealand as Part of a Rapid Response to the COVID-19 Pandemic,"[63] the University of Otago stated, "the paper published by

[63] Rhodri Harfoot, et al., "Characterization of the First SARS-CoV-2 Isolates from Aotearoa New Zealand as Part of a Rapid Response to the COVID-19 Pandemic", *Viruses,* 10 Feb 2022: https://doi.org/10.3390/v14020366

Professor Quiñones-Mateu and colleagues was a descriptive paper...This means there was no hypothesis to prove or disprove."[64] In a nutshell, the response perhaps unwittingly summarised the wider state of affairs in virology. In 2008, the journal *Infection and Immunity* featured a guest commentary titled, "Descriptive Science" that explained why, "descriptive research by itself is seldom conclusive," and may simply serve as a starting point to orientate further investigations.[65] The authors pointed out that, "microbiology and immunology are now experimental sciences and consequently investigators can go beyond simply describing observations to formulate hypotheses and then perform experiments to validate or refute them." As this essay outlines, the virology establishment will not divulge or carry out these required experiments, seemingly in order not to refute itself. It intentionally limits itself to ongoing opportunistic fishing-expeditions backed by confirmation bias, thus disqualifying itself from the scientific method due to its inconsistency with the hypothesis-driven and falsifiable approach described by Popper.

The author has previously written in a postscript derived from A. F. Chalmers' book *What is this thing called Science?*, that one of the pivotal issues with virology was that it invented itself as a field before establishing if viruses actually existed. It has been trying to justify itself since its inception:

> *In this instance, a virus particle was not observed first and subsequently viral theory and pathology developed. Scientists of the mid and late nineteenth century were preoccupied with the identification of imagined contagious pathogenic entities.*

---

[64] Letter from Kelsey Kennard, University of Otago, "Official information request for information regarding the paper 'Characterization of the First SARS-CoV-2 Isolates from Aotearoa New Zealand as Part of a Rapid Response to the COVID-19 Pandemic'", 22 Jun 2022.

[65] Arturo Casadevall and Ferric Fang, "Descriptive Science", *Infection and Immunity*, 14 Jul 2008: https://doi.org/10.1128/iai.00743-08

> *The observations of the naïve inductionist did not identify a virus* a priori, *and then set about studying its properties and characteristics. The extant presupposition of the time was that a very small germ particle existed that may explain contagion. What came thereafter arose to fulfil the presuppositional premise.*[66]

Because a scientific theory demands evidence that has repeatedly been tested and corroborated in accordance with the scientific method, it is clear that "viruses" never even reached the stage of a theory.[67] According to the science, they remain mere speculation.

VIROLOGY'S LACK OF CONTROLS MEANS IT IS NOT A SCIENTIFIC PURSUIT

OIA requests have revealed that New Zealand's Institute of Environmental Science and Research (ESR), who have claimed isolation and genomic sequencing of the SARS-CoV-2 particle in the Antipodes, are also guilty of failing to perform any valid controls.[68] In the tradition of Enders, they have not paused to check whether the CPEs they witnessed, or genomes they assembled via computer simulations, could also be created in valid control comparisons. That is, by performing experiments with other human-derived specimens, from both well subjects and unwell subjects who are said not to have the alleged disease COVID-19. Instead, ESR described their insufficient "negative control" in which, "the flask undergoes the same conditions as the flasks used for viral culture, however we use Infection media only."

---

[66] Mark Bailey, "Warnings Signs You Have Been Tricked By Virologists...Again", 25 Jul 2022: https://drsambailey.com/warnings-signs-you-have-been-tricked-by-virologists-again/

[67] Ibid.

[68] Mark Bailey, "Fact-check: New Zealand can't find the 'SARS-CoV-2 virus'", 12 Feb 2022: https://drsambailey.com/covid-19/fact-check-new-zealand-cant-find-the-sars-cov-2-virus/

The central conductor in these anti-scientific pursuits is the WHO. It is very telling that in their 94-page "Genomic sequencing of SARS-CoV-2" document, there is a mere four sentences discussing "control samples:"

> *6.4.2 Control samples*
>
> *Negative control samples, such as buffer or water, should always be included in any sequencing run that contains multiple samples. They should be included at the earliest stage possible and should proceed with samples through all stages of the sequencing pipeline. This is extremely important to rule out contamination during a sequencing run that occurs in the laboratory or during bioinformatic processing.*
>
> *Positive control samples with known genetic sequences can be useful to validate newly adopted or adapted bioinformatic pipelines for consensus calling, but do not need to be included in every sequencing run.*[69]

However, neither of these controls are sufficient to validate the "genomes" that the virologists are producing through these techniques because they can only serve to calibrate the pipeline. As has become apparent, the WHO cannot point to one valid positive control experiment, yet on February 11, 2020 they named the new disease they had invented, "COVID-19" with the associated claim that it was caused by a novel coronavirus.[70] They have provided the green light for anyone around the world to "find" SARS-CoV-2 in their backyards without the need for valid control experiments either. Yet, there is a clear necessity for comparative controls where similar patient samples, but without the alleged virus, are processed in the same way so that only one variable is being tested.

[69] World Health Organization, "Genomic sequencing of SARS-CoV-2 - A guide to implementation for maximum impact on public health", 8 Jan 2021.

[70] "WHO Director-General's remarks at the media briefing on 2019-nCoV on 11 February 2020", WHO, 11 Feb 2020: https://www.who.int/director-general/speeches/detail/who-director-general-s-remarks-at-the-media-briefing-on-2019-ncov-on-11-february-2020

Comparing the results of a sample alleged to contain the virus with one of the negative controls described by the WHO's document above cannot validate the process as the latter samples do not contain the genetic soup that is part of the former. In any case, even on their own terms the negative control referred to by ESR in New Zealand is unable to provide validation of the methodology they are using to create these virus genomes, because as the WHO states, it is simply a precautionary check for contamination.

With all of the failures to culture postulated viruses, modern virology now favours direct metagenomics[71] of crude samples, often with shotgun sequencing[72] and subsequent artificial assembly of these genetic fragments to create new *in silico*[73] "viruses" out of thin air. This invention then provides other virus hunters with predesigned PCR primer panels[74] so that they can also discover the same sequences and claim it is the same virus. ESR were involved in a publication in which they proclaimed the discovery of SARS-CoV-2 in nine subjects through this methodology.[75] They

---

71 "Metagenomics is the study of the structure and function of entire nucleotide sequences isolated and analyzed from all the organisms (typically microbes) in a bulk sample. Metagenomics is often used to study a specific community of microorganisms, such as those residing on human skin, in the soil or in a water sample." - NIH National Human Genome Research Institute, "Metagenomics": https://www.genome.gov/genetics-glossary/Metagenomics (accessed 27 Apr 2022). It is an illegitimate methodology when used by virologists as none of the sequences that are obtained and declared to be "viral" have been shown to come from a virus at any time as this essay will detail.

72 Shotgun sequencing is a method that randomly fragments the DNA in a sample into short segments, for example 150 base pairs in length. These short fragments are sequenced to obtain "reads". From this point the process relies on sequence assembly software to arrange overlapping reads into "contigs".

73 "In or on a computer: done or produced by using computer software or simulation.": https://www.merriam-webster.com/dictionary/in%20silico

74 Example for SARS-CoV-2: "xGen™ SARS-CoV-2 Amplicon Panels": https://sg.idtdna.com/pages/products/next-generation-sequencing/workflow/xgen-ngs-amplicon-sequencing/predesigned-amplicon-panels/sars-cov-2-amp-panel

75 Nick Eichler, et al., "Transmission of severe acute respiratory syndrome coronavirus 2 during border quarantine and air travel, New Zealand (Aotearoa)", *Emerg Infect Dis.*, May 2021: https://doi.org/10.3201/eid2705.210514

were asked by my colleague to provide, "all details of the control group that was used when comparing the results of sequencing," but instead of answering the question, the ESR made an excuse about not getting involved in the "generation of new data," and provided some links to SARS-CoV-2 sequencing protocols.[76] If ESR were using such protocols, as detailed on the protocol.io site, then we can see that they are endorsing insufficient controls that are described as, "[a] negative control of nuclease-free water," while an optional "positive control can also be included which may be a synthetic RNA constructs or high-titre clinical sample which can be diluted."[77] Once again, these types of controls can only serve as pipeline calibration techniques, not the validation or the clinical significance of any "genomes" they assemble.

Despite the resources available to them, ESR apparently do not believe in the necessity to check for themselves whether SARS-CoV-2 can be shown to exist. On 19 July 2022, in response to an OIA request they stated that, "ESR has not performed any experiments to scientifically prove the existence of SARS-COV-2 virus and can therefore not provide you with any records."[78] On 17 August 2022 in response to another request, they admitted that, "ESR has not performed any experiments to scientifically prove that [the] SARS-COV-2 virus causes COVID-19 and can therefore not provide you with any records."[79] Nobody else has performed these required scientific experiments either.

---

76 (Letter from ESR, 'Official Information Act Request: OIA Request for records from doi: 10.3201/eid2705.210514', 25 Mar 2022.)

77 protocols.io, "nCoV-2019 sequencing protocol v3 (LoCost) V.3": https://www.protocols.io/view/ncov-2019-sequencing-protocol-v3-locost-bp2l6n26rgqe/v3?step=1 (accessed 28 Mar 2022).

78 (Letter from ESR, 'Official Information Act Request: FOIA: SARS-CoV-2 Proof of Existence', 19 Jul 2022.)

79 Letter from ESR, 'Official Information Act Request: SARS-CoV-2 Proof of Causation', 17 Aug 2022: https://www.fluoridefreepeel.ca/wp-content/uploads/2022/09/2022-08-29-ESR-SARS-COV-2-Proof-of-Causation-Redacted.pdf

ANIMAL ABUSE AND "ANTIBODY" STUDIES

With the inability to demonstrate the physical isolation of a disease-causing particle that meets the definition of a virus, the virologists have engaged in animal experiments to convince the uninitiated that such pathogenic particles exist. The hallmark of these publications is that they lack valid controls, so even on the unestablished premise that they are handling "viruses," they reveal another aspect of virology's anti-science. An illustrative example was the paper, "Comparative pathogenesis of COVID-19, MERS, and SARS in a nonhuman primate model," published in May 2020 by a team that included Christian Drosten and Ron Fouchier.[80] The nonsense of what was published in *Science* can be summarised as follows:

1. The eight cynomolgus monkeys in the experiments were, *"inoculated with SARS-CoV-2 under anesthesia via a combination of intratracheal (4.5 ml) and intranasal (0.25 ml per nostril) routes..."*[81] — This is not a natural exposure route and 4.5ml poured into a small (3.5 - 5.0kg) monkey's lungs is equivalent to pouring around 80ml (⅓ cup) of foreign biological material into a human's lungs, while they are asleep. This volume of material alone is enough to cause damage and inflammation in the lung tissue.
2. The inoculum poured into their lungs was made from, "SARS-CoV-2 (isolate BetaCoV/Munich/BavPat1/2020) obtained from a clinical case in Germany," and, "the virus was propagated to passage three on Vero E6 cells in Opti-MEM I (1X) + GlutaMAX (Gibco), supplemented with penicillin (10,000 IU/mL) and streptomycin (10,000 IU/mL)." — They have asserted that they have a viral 'isolate' when neither they nor

[80] Barry Rockx, et al., "Comparative pathogenesis of COVID-19, MERS, and SARS in a nonhuman primate model", Science, 29 May 2020: https://www.science.org/doi/10.1126/science.abb7314

[81] Ibid, supplementary material.

their supplier[82] have demonstrated the existence of a virus in the sample. All that can be said is that the sample contains foreign biological material from the human-derived clinical specimen and monkey kidney cells, in addition to cellular breakdown products and two antibiotics.

3. "No overt clinical signs were observed in any of the infected animals, except for a serous nasal discharge in one aged animal on day 14 post inoculation (p.i.). No significant weight loss was observed in any of the animals during the study." — In other words, despite the direct entry into the lungs with what they claimed was the SARS-CoV-2 virus, it didn't make any of the monkeys noticeably sick.
4. "By day 14 p.i., all remaining animals seroconverted as revealed by the presence of SARS-CoV-2–specific antibodies against the virus S1 domain and nucleocapsid proteins in their sera." — The S1 and nucleocapsid proteins have not been shown to be viral in origin regardless of whether they induce the detection (through an *in vitro* assay) of other proteins termed "antibodies" in a host. The virologists once again employ circular reasoning to claim that the detection of an antibody proves the existence of a virus because the antibody is declared to be specific to the alleged virus.
5. "As a measure of virus shedding, nasal, throat, and rectal swabs were assayed for virus by reverse transcription–quantitative polymerase chain reaction (RT-qPCR)..." — There was no "virus shedding," there was simply detection of the same sequences that had been recently poured into the monkeys' respiratory tracts. These foreign nucleic acid sequences unsurprisingly disappeared from the monkeys' bodies over the next few days through natural clearance mechanisms.
6. "SARS-CoV-2 RNA was only detected in a rectal swab from one animal on day 14 p.i., and no viral RNA was detected in whole blood at any time point throughout the study." — Again this indicates that they were only finding the introduced genetic material in the same places

[82] European Virus Archive Global, "Human 2019-nCoV Isolate": https://www.european-virus-archive.com/virus/human-2019-ncov-isolate

it had been introduced. (The single positive rectal swab may have been a false positive or the monkey had swallowed some of the introduced biological material.) In not one case could they demonstrate that the postulated "virus" had any invasive characteristics.

7. Four of the monkeys were killed and autopsied 4 days after inoculation with the foreign biological soup. Two out of the four were reported as having small foci of consolidation in their lungs, and the authors stated that, "the main histological lesion in the consolidated pulmonary tissues of both the young and aged animals involved the alveoli and bronchioles and consisted of areas with acute or more advanced DAD [diffuse alveolar damage]." The histological features were asserted to be characteristic of 'SARS-CoV-2' — see Figure 3 below for an explanation of why these claims are completely baseless.
8. "SARS-CoV-2 antigen expression was detected in moderate numbers of type I pneumocytes and a few type II pneumocytes within foci of DAD." — This was claimed through an immunohistochemistry (IHC) staining technique that was based on, "a rabbit polyclonal antibody against SARS-CoV-nucleoprotein (40143-T62, Sino Biological, Chesterbrook, PA, USA)." Unfortunately for them the supplier of this product states, "IHC, FCM, IF, IP et al. applications haven't been validated. (Antibody's applications haven't been validated with corresponding virus positive samples.)"[83] In any case, this example can be used to expose the wider fallacy regarding antibodies as "evidence" of viruses. Sino Biological states that the antibodies were the result of injecting their "SARS-CoV Nucleocapsid Protein (His Tag)" product[84] into rabbits. This nucleocapsid protein was in turn produced from, "a DNA sequence encoding the SARS-CoV (isolate:Tor2) nucleoprotein." We will see on page 30 that the "Tor2" sequence was

---

83 "SARS-CoV/SARS-CoV-2 Nucleocapsid Antibody, Rabbit PAb, Antigen Affinity Purified", Sino Biological: https://www.sinobiological.com/antibodies/cov-nucleocapsid-40143-t62

84 "SARS-CoV Nucleocapsid Protein (His Tag)", Sino Biological: https://www.sinobiological.com/recombinant-proteins/sars-cov-nucleocapsid-40143-v08b

one of the two *in silico* templates used by Fan Wu et al. to invent SARS-CoV-2, another *in silico* model. In summary, it engages in more circular reasoning: no protein has been shown to come from a virus, including the nucleocapsid protein in this case. It was simply asserted that they injected "viral" proteins into animals and in response the animals produced other proteins that are claimed to be "antibodies." However, a virus was neither shown to exist, nor required to exist for this sort of exercise. (As another example, the generation of "HIV antibodies" in 100% of healthy volunteers injected with a University of Queensland COVID-19 candidate vaccine stands out as an embarrassment for those promulgating both the HIV and antibody industries.[85])

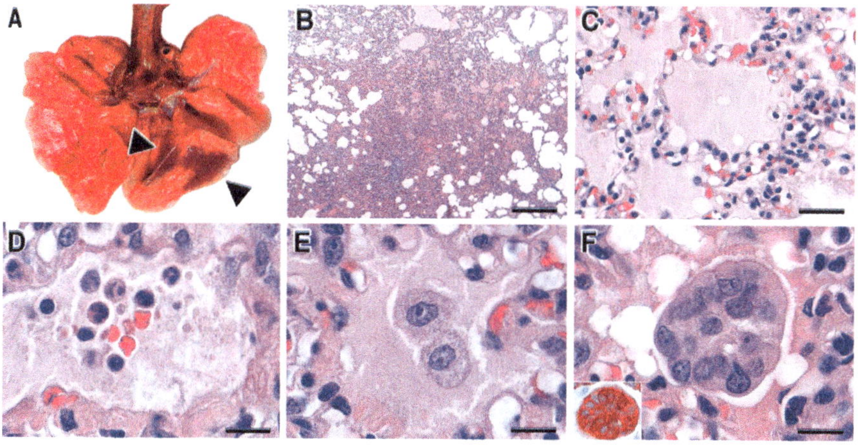

Figure 3. Some of the images presented in the "Comparative pathogenesis of COVID-19, MERS, and SARS in a nonhuman primate model" paper and claimed to be, "characteristic pathological changes," of SARS-CoV-2. The lung changes in (A)-(C) are consistent with pneumonitis, caused by pouring a liquid containing foreign biological material directly into the monkey's trachea while it was anaesthetised. The histological changes (D)-(F) simply depict inflammatory cells such as macrophages and neutrophils as would be expected in such an inflicted pneumonitis. No control experiments were performed.

[85] Dr Sam Bailey, "Covid-19 Shots, Cancer and HIV", 14 Jul 2021: https://drsambailey.com/resources/videos/vaccines/covid-19-shots-cancer-and-hiv/

However, the most flawed aspect of the animal experiment was that it did not follow the scientific method as it lacked controls. That is, a comparable group of monkeys was not subjected to an internal assault with the same composition and volume of biological soup, *sans* the alleged "virus," being poured directly into their lungs. To be clear, the author does not endorse such an experiment as it is a cruel procedure that has nothing to do with natural exposure routes — it is simply to point out the concept of an adequately controlled experiment. Unfortunately, such unscientific methodologies are sadly replicated in all such animal studies that have been reviewed. Not one of them demonstrates: (a) a natural method of exposure utilising the samples alleged to contain viruses, (b) valid "mock-infections" (for example, the disingenuous use of phosphate-buffered saline only), or (c) animal-to-animal *disease* transmission. That is of course in addition to the foundational issue that none of the studies show the actual existence of an infectious particle they are purporting to test.

Additionally, if the "viruses" are so infectious, why not simply aerosolise a sample into the animal cages so they inhale it? Once again such experiments are avoided in order for the virologists not to refute themselves with regard to claims of contagion involving the imagined particles.

THE VIRUS QUANTITY PARADOX

We are led to believe that inside a host such as a human, the viral particles are produced in such great numbers that they can rupture the very cells containing them, while at the same time they are present in such tiny amounts that virologists say they can't be seen in any patient specimens. Apparently with regard to the alleged SARS-CoV-2 particle it has been calculated that, "one sneeze of a COVID-19 patient contains 200 million viruses."[86] However, if we obtain a (physically larger) sample directly from a subject's nose or lungs there are precisely none to be found. To cover up this inconvenient problem, the virologists have resorted to proffering indirect "evidence" through tissue cultures in an attempt to pull the missing virus out of the hat. As we outlined in *The COVID-19 Fraud & War on Humanity*, this involves the second part of virology's *double deception* which is, "the substitution of the fake proxy of inducing cytopathic effects (CPEs) by inoculating typically abnormal cell lines *in vitro* for the postulated proxy of infecting a healthy or non-diseased host *in vivo* to establish causality between the purported pathogen and the disease."[87] So we are supposed to believe that the human respiratory tract, which is lined with the alleged perfect host cells, does not produce enough viruses for them to be seen, but a test tube experiment involving tissue from a different species and cell type does?

By virology's definition the hypothesised particles are passive and do not produce any waste products so it is thus a mystery as to how they inflict ill health on a human host. Pfizer suggested to the layperson that, "the immune system reacts to the injury of these bodily cells by revving up," but did not cite any scientific evidence for this imaginative claim.[88] The 4th edition of *Medical Microbiology* ventured further and stated that:

> *Direct cell damage and death from viral infection* ***may*** *result from (1) diversion of the cell's energy, (2) shutoff of cell macromolecular synthesis, (3) competition of viral mRNA for cellular ribosomes, (4) competition of viral promoters and*

---

[86] "Number of the day: one sneeze of a COVID-19 patient contains 200 million viruses", *Новые известия*, 22 May 2020: https://en.newizv.ru/news/science/22-05-2020/digit-of-the-day-200-million-viruses-are-contained-in-one-sneeze-of-a-patient-of-covid-19

[87] Mark Bailey & John Bevan-Smith, "The COVID-19 Fraud & War on Humanity", 11 Nov 2021: https://drsambailey.com/covid-19/the-covid-19-fraud-war-on-humanity/

[88] "How do Viruses Make us Sick?", *Pfizer.com*: https://www.pfizer.com/news/articles/how_do_viruses_make_us_sick (accessed 20 May 2022).

> *transcriptional enhancers for cellular transcriptional factors such as RNA polymerases, and inhibition of the interferon defense mechanisms. Indirect cell damage can result from integration of the viral genome, induction of mutations in the host genome, inflammation, and the host immune response.*[89] [My emphasis.]

Essentially, the virologists have offered multiple *hypothetical* pathogenetic mechanisms for a particle hypothesised to exist in an organism such as a human. And again, even if these speculative mechanisms were at play, it would require *enormous* numbers of cells to be affected to produce symptoms. But enormous numbers of cells would result in astronomical amounts of viral particles coming out of them — so why can no viral particles ever be found? Virology has a habit of diverting attention away from such aspects that raise doubts about its phantasmal model.

---

[89] Samuel Baron, et al., "Viral Pathogenesis" in *Medical Microbiology*, 4th edition, 1996: https://www.ncbi.nlm.nih.gov/books/NBK8149/

PART TWO

FAN WU ET AL. DEUS EX MACHINA

They were bound to, determined to find a virus as the cause for this guy. So they did this dragnet for all of this RNA, millions of little strands of RNA in this person, using technology that's called meta-transcriptomics. And its one of these gene things...they can look at all the RNA, all the DNA, sequence it, amplify it... It's technology driven, not science driven...And they came up with a sequence and then they decided that they had discovered a "virus", even though they never touched a virus at all, and they said that was the cause of this guy's pneumonia.

— Dr David Rasnick, on the "discovery" of SARS-CoV-2 by Fan Wu et al.[90]

In *The COVID-19 Fraud & War on Humanity*[91] we documented the invention of SARS-CoV-2 by Fan Wu's team who assembled an *in silico* "genome" from genetic fragments of unknown provenance, found in the crude lung washings of a single 'case' and documented in, "A new coronavirus associated with human respiratory disease in China."[92] A further analysis of this paper is indicated as it illustrates how the fraudulent COVID-19 pandemic was created by means of an invented "genome" through deep meta-transcriptomic sequencing, which simply sought to detect all the RNA in a crude sample, and how it was misused to invent a non-existent pathogen. The claim that anyone can declare,

[90] "Episode One: The Tragic Pseudoscience of SARS-CoV-2", *The Viral Delusion*, Paradigm Shift, 2022: https://paradigmshift.uscreen.io/

[91] Mark Bailey & John Bevan-Smith, "The COVID-19 Fraud & War on Humanity", 11 Nov 2021: https://drsambailey.com/covid-19/the-covid-19-fraud-war-on-humanity/

[92] Fan Wu, et al., "A new coronavirus associated with human respiratory disease in China", *Nature*, 579, 265–269, 3 Feb 2020: https://doi.org/10.1038/s41586-020-2008-3

"[they] identified a new RNA virus strain from the family *Coronaviridae*, which is designated here 'WH-Human 1' coronavirus,"[93] from a *single* human subject diagnosed with pneumonia is farcical in itself. The authors tried to justify this by stating, "although the isolation of the virus from only a single patient is not sufficient to conclude that it caused these respiratory symptoms, our findings have been independently corroborated in further patients in a separate study." Firstly, there was no physical isolation of any virus as will be discussed in detail momentarily. Secondly, their claim of being "independently corroborated" is a reference to the February 2020 paper of Peng Zhou et al. — a paper that cannot corroborate anything and the fraud of which is discussed on page 41. All that can be said is that if circular reasoning is employed, then finding similar genetic sequences on more than one occasion is seen as confirmation of a virus. The GISAID database is the treasure chest of this virological nonsense and by 29 August 2022 had over 12.8 million claims of having 'found' SARS-CoV-2.[94] However none of them can point to an actual virus, they are simply calling 'bingo' by assembling similar sequences which they have aligned with Fan Wu et al. and other previous assemblies, no actual virus required.

It should also be noted that while the author does not make pronouncement as to the *cause* of any case of pneumonia or acute febrile respiratory syndromes, the general medical community acknowledges that no "pathogen" is identified in around half of the cases.[95,96] So what reason did Fan Wu et al. have to suspect that their patient was harbouring a brand new virus? Apparently because, "epidemiological investigations by

---

93 Ibid.

94 GISAID: https://www.gisaid.org/ (accessed 29 Aug 2022).

95 Catia Cilloniz, et al., "Microbial Etiology of Pneumonia: Epidemiology, Diagnosis and Resistance Patterns", *Int. J. Mol. Sci.*, 17(12), 2120, 16 Dec 2016.

96 Gao Liu, et al., "Viral and Bacterial Etiology of Acute Febrile Respiratory Syndrome among Patients in Qinghai, China", *Biomed Environ Sci*, Jun 2019: https://www.besjournal.com/article/doi/10.3967/bes2019.058

the Wuhan Center for Disease Control and Prevention revealed that the patient worked at a local indoor seafood market."[97] It would seem a very weak reason given the fact that these wet markets are extremely common in China and that despite the bat-origin theories, Fan Wu et al. reported, "no bats were available for sale."

In any case, they obtained some bronchoalveolar lavage fluid (BALF) from their patient and with this crude specimen reported that, "total RNA was extracted from 200µl of BALF." Their methods section detailed that this was achieved, "using the RNeasy Plus Universal Mini kit (Qiagen)," i.e. through spin column centrifugation. They claimed that, "ribosomal RNA depletion was performed during library construction," however, see page 62 as to why this is dubious as there remained a high match for known human RNA sequences. They then proceeded to shotgun sequence the brew, starting with random fragmentation of the genetic material into short lengths averaging 150 nucleotides and conversion of the RNA to DNA using a reverse transcriptase enzyme.[98] 56,565,928 such short reads were generated and this information was fed into Megahit and Trinity, software platforms for *de novo* algorithm-based assembly. Through Megahit, 384,096 contigs, or hypothetical overlapping sequences were generated and the longest one (30,474 nucleotides) was declared to have a "nucleotide identity of 89.1%" to bat SL-CoVZC45, another fictional construct that will be dealt with subsequently. (Trinity generated over 1.3 million contigs but the longest one was only 11,760 nucleotides — in other words, they would not have found the "genome" if they had just used this software platform.) The word 'virus' suddenly appeared when they state, "the genome sequence of this virus, as well as its termini, were determined and confirmed by reverse-transcription PCR." This is a sleight

---

[97] Fan Wu, et al., "A new coronavirus associated with human respiratory disease in China", *Nature,* 579, 265–269, 3 Feb 2020: https://doi.org/10.1038/s41586-020-2008-3

[98] Illumina, "RNA Sequencing Methods Collection", 2017: https://www.illumina.com/content/dam/illumina-marketing/documents/products/research_reviews/rna-sequencing-methods-review-web.pdf

of hand as the PCR simply amplifies pre-selected sequences and has no capacity to confirm a previously unknown genome. As PCR expert Stephen Bustin has explained, "PCR requires you to know what the sequence of your target is...so once you know that there's something in your sample, then you would try to isolate it, yes. And then once you've isolated it, then you sequence it again, or PCR it up."[99] In other words, PCR itself cannot identify the origins of the sequences and the methodology of Fan Wu et al. did not establish the origin of their described sequences. However, in the very next sentence they announce to the world that, "this virus strain was designated as WH-Human 1 coronavirus (WHCV)".

> — *We need to pause at this point as it is where the fraudulent virus, soon to be renamed SARS-CoV-2,* ***was invented out of thin air.*** *A virus that the WHO claims, with no evidential support whatsoever, is the causative agent of COVID-19.*

For it is this "genome" that was submitted to GenBank on the 5th of January 2020[100] that was seized on by Drosten et al. to help produce their phoney PCR protocol assay sequences,[101] which in turn were published with indecent haste by the WHO for all the world to use, thereby turning WH-Human 1 into the world's reference genome for a claimed pathogen. It is this invention that is responsible for the whole bag of destructive

---

[99] *Planet Waves FM* with Eric F. Coppolino, "Interview with Dr. Stephen Bustin", 1 Feb 2021: https://planetwaves.net/planet-waves-fm-interview-with-dr-stephen-bustin/, transcript by Joshua Halinen: https://cormandrostenreview.com/wp-content/uploads/2021/02/bustin-transcript.pdf

[100] Zhang, et al., "Wuhan seafood market pneumonia virus isolate Wuhan-Hu-1, complete genome, GenBank: MN908947.1", submitted 5 Jan 2020: https://www.ncbi.nlm.nih.gov/nuccore/MN908947.1

[101] Victor Corman and Christian Drosten, et al., "Detection of 2019 novel coronavirus (2019-nCoV) by real-time RT-PCR", *Euro Surveill*, 23 Jan 2020: https://doi.org/10.2807/1560-7917.ES.2020.25.3.2000045. In addition to GenBank: MN908947.1, that was first made publicly available at virological.org (https://virological.org/t/novel-2019-coronavirus-genome/319), Drosten et al. also employed "four other genomes deposited on 12 January in the viral sequence database curated by the Global Initiative on Sharing All Influenza Data (GISAID)," in designing their PCR protocols.

tricks imposed on the world following the announcement of the pandemic by the WHO on the 11th of March 2020.[102]

However, anyone paying attention can see that there is no evidence whatsoever of a virus in the Fan Wu et al. paper. A virus is claimed to be a tiny replication-competent obligate intracellular parasite, consisting of a genome surrounded by a proteinaceous coat: it is an infectious particle that *causes* disease in a host. All Fan Wu et al. had was a 41-year-old man with pneumonia and a software-assembled model "genome" made from sequences of unestablished origin found in the man's lung washings. To make it appear legitimate they stated, "the viral genome organization of WHCV was determined by sequence alignment to two representative members of the genus Betacoronavirus: a coronavirus associated with humans (SARS-CoV Tor2, GenBank accession number AY274119) and a coronavirus associated with bats (bat SL-CoVZC45, GenBank accession number MG772933)." These alleged genomes are also simply *in silico* constructs that have never been proven to exist in their entirety in nature, let alone been shown to come from inside a virus. For example bat SL-CoVZC45 was invented in 2018 by the process of, "19 degenerated PCR primer pairs...designed by multiple alignment of available SARS-CoV and bat SL-CoV sequences deposited in GenBank."[103]

The virus genomes have become what is possibly the greatest illusion in virology, an illusion which propagates a belief that viruses are indeed being shown to exist. The virologists themselves don't seem to appreciate the fatal flaw in their methodologies even when they state it themselves:

> *Three main methods based on HTS [high-throughput sequencing] are currently used for viral whole-genome*

---

[102] WHO, "WHO Director-General's opening remarks at the media briefing on COVID-19 - 11 March 2020", 11 Mar 2020.

[103] Dan Hu, et al. "Genomic characterization and infectivity of a novel SARS-like coronavirus in Chinese bats", *Emerging microbes & infections,* 12 Sep 2018: https://doi.org/10.1038/s41426-018-0155-5

> *sequencing: metagenomic sequencing, target enrichment sequencing and PCR amplicon sequencing, each showing benefits and drawbacks (Houldcroft et al., 2017). In metagenomic sequencing, total DNA (and/or RNA) from a sample including host but also bacteria, viruses and fungi is extracted and sequenced. It is a simple and cost-effective approach, and it is the only approach not requiring reference sequences. Instead, the other two HTS approaches, target enrichment and amplicon sequencing, both depend on reference information to design baits or primers. The limitation of metagenomic sequencing is that it requires a very high sequencing depth to obtain enough viral genome material.*[104]

The more important limitation with 'viral' sequencing is that the process itself does not determine the provenance of the genetic fragments, so how can it be used to establish the sequence of a previously unknown genome? For clarity, we are not talking about situations where the provenance of the sequences can be independently verified, for example, physically-isolated bacterial cells. Additionally, it is nonsensical to arbitrarily declare that sequences are viral by a process of elimination, that is, based on the fact that they do not have a previously conflicting assignation on the genetic databanks. None of the virologists are demonstrating that the sequences are viral in nature when they assemble the very first template and declare they have discovered a pathogenic virus. At no stage are any of them purifying alleged viral particles to prove their relationship with the sequences. And yet the first invented *de novo* genome becomes the touchstone with which other virus hunters will align their own *in silico* genomes or design 'confirmatory' PCR protocols.

---

[104] Florence Maurier, et al., "A complete protocol for whole-genome sequencing of virus from clinical samples: Application to coronavirus OC43", *Virology*, 531, May 2019: https://doi.org/10.1016/j.virol.2019.03.006

As far as the author is aware, the virologists do not have any laboratory techniques that can directly check whether there even exists a complete 30 kilobase RNA strand in any of their samples. Existing pulsed-field gel electrophoresis technology can only reliably differentiate *DNA* strands of this size.[105] In any case, these simulations remain a distraction because even in the event that the physical existence of an *in silico* SARS-CoV-2 genome — a complete 30 kilobase RNA sequence — can be shown to exist in nature, the virologists would still have plenty of work to do. First and foremost they would have to demonstrate that this sequence belongs to a *disease-causing* replication-competent particle that can make a person ill and not just *claim* it does.

On that note, the author had an email exchange with an evolutionary biologist from the Wellcome Sanger Institute who suggested that long-read RNA sequencing (as opposed to only shotgun sequencing) provided the necessary proof of the existence of "SARS-CoV-2".[106] He referred to an April 2022 publication involving RNA-sequencing through Oxford Nanopore Technologies (ONT) long-reads,[107] claiming that it confirmed the validity of the "virus" genomes that had been previously constructed through shotgun sequencing. The proffered study described an experiment comparing responses between various "SARS-CoV-2-infected" and "mock-infected" cell-lines. The experimental cells were alleged to be "infected with SARS-CoV-2 Australia virus (Australia/VIC01/2020, NCBI: MT007544.1)" — claimed by author Leon Caly et al. to be an "isolate",[108]

---

[105] David Schwartz and Charles Cantor, "Separation of Yeast Chromosome-Sized DNAs by Pulsed Field Gradient Gel Electrophoresis", *Cell*, Vol. 37, May 1984: https://doi.org/10.1016/0092-8674(84)90301-5

[106] By email from Zachary Ardern: https://www.fluoridefreepeel.ca/wp-content/uploads/2022/06/Mark-Bailey-Zachary-Ardern-emails-redacted.pdf

[107] Jessie Chang, et al., "Long-Read RNA Sequencing Identifies Polyadenylation Elongation and Differential Transcript Usage of Host Transcripts During SARS-CoV-2 In Vitro Infection", *Front. Immunol.*, 6 April 2022: https://doi.org/10.3389/fimmu.2022.832223

[108] Leon Caly, et al., "Isolation and rapid sharing of the 2019 novel coronavirus (SARS-CoV-2) from the first patient diagnosed with COVID-19 in Australia", *Med. J. Aust.*, 1 Apr 2020: https://doi.org/10.5694/mja2.50569

when isolation of a virus was never demonstrated, as explained in Figure 4 below, and as we outlined in *The COVID-19 Fraud & War on Humanity.*[109] Hence, the evolutionary biologist's argument relied on the fraudulent product of a fraudulent experiment being compared with a "mock-infection," where the former is invalidated by the misleading declaration of "virus isolation" and the latter invalidates itself as the virologists have changed its definition to allow other variables to be altered. Obtaining longer reads does not change these foundational issues. The evolutionary biologist was asserting that variations in monitored sequences and proteins over time represented evidence of an evolving virus.[110] He is another victim of virology's deception through their specious attachment of the word 'viral' to these entities. When all such sequences and proteins

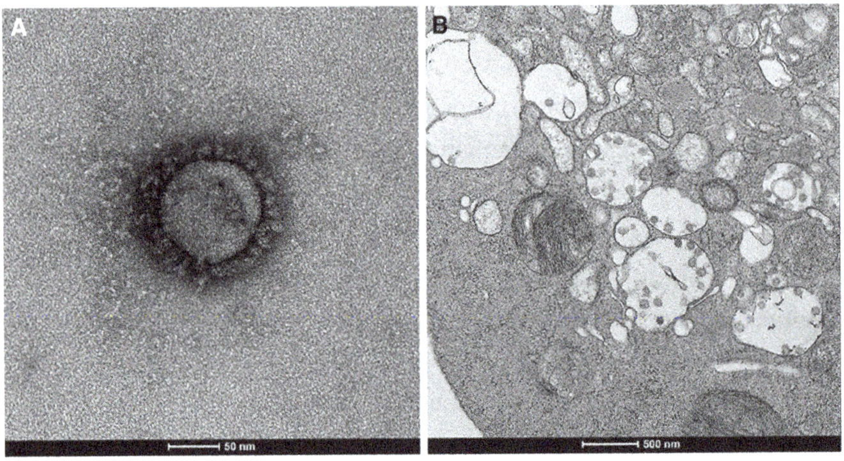

Figure 4. Caly et al. "isolation" of SARS-CoV-2. The electron micrographs are of a Vero/hSLAM cell culture supernatant: (A) was declared to be a "virion", when it is simply a particle of unknown provenance. Additionally, the capsular 'spikes' were produced *after* the enzyme trypsin digested the outer proteins to create the desired appearance. (B) simply informs us the size of the particles in a mixture of tissue. There was no valid control experiment performed with a similar human-derived specimen.

109 Mark Bailey & John Bevan-Smith, "The COVID-19 Fraud & War on Humanity", 11 Nov 2021: https://drsambailey.com/covid-19/the-covid-19-fraud-war-on-humanity/

110 By email from Zachary Ardern: https://www.fluoridefreepeel.ca/wp-content/uploads/2022/06/Mark-Bailey-Zachary-Ardern-emails-redacted.pdf

were originally detected in tissue culture experiments they were not shown to belong to pathogenic viruses but the claim that they are "viral" continues to this day.

Along the same lines and a few months after that exchange, the pathologist/virologist Dr Sin Hang Lee claimed that his preprint paper[111] provided, "irrefutable Sanger sequencing evidence that the virus [SARS-CoV-2] exists and keeps mutating," with an open invitation to challenge his work.[112] Again, the present author provided a response, detailing virology's ongoing misuse of scientific terminology as well as the underlying problem of unestablished provenance of the genetic sequences being analysed:

> *To expose the problems of virology it is crucial to examine the methodology section of any publication and in this case it is no different...Those of us that dispute the virus narrative point out that no RNA (or DNA) sequences have ever been shown to come from inside any specific identifiable particle that fulfils the definition of a virus. Thus all RNAs can only be said to be expressed by a known organism, introduced artificially (e.g. synthetic mRNA injections) or be of unknown provenance. The "mutations" only exist within* in silico *models that have not been shown to be independent entities in nature. There are other reasons why RNA sequences can and do vary in dynamic biological systems and I can't imagine that any virologist would disagree with this fact. Simply detecting RNAs is not enough to draw conclusions about their provenance. Other experiments are required to make this determination.*[113]

[111] Sin Lee, " Implementation of the eCDC/WHO Recommendation for Molecular Diagnosis of SARS-CoV-2 Omicron Subvariants and Its Challenges", *preprints.org*, 14 Jun 2022: https://www.preprints.org/manuscript/202206.0192/v1

[112] Mark Bailey, "Warnings Signs You Have Been Tricked By Virologists...Again", 25 Jul 2022: https://drsambailey.com/warnings-signs-you-have-been-tricked-by-virologists-again/

[113] Ibid.

Indeed, no amount of genomic or proteomic technology can escape the fact that with regard to such data being supposed evidence of viruses, it is turtles all the way down.

TURTLES ALL THE WAY DOWN

As has been noted, 'bat SL-CoVZC45' was an *in silico* genome, 29,802 nucleotides in length, invented in 2018,[114] that was used by Fan Wu et al. as a template genome for the invention of the SARS-CoV-2 genome. It was purported to come from the intestinal tissue of a bat that was captured in Zhejiang province, China. In this study the authors reported that, "all bats appeared healthy and had no obvious clinical signs at capture," but declared that a virus was detected in 89 out of 334 bats on the basis of a, "pan-coronavirus reverse transcription (RT)-PCR assay." The folly of claiming 'isolation' of any virus through inducing CPEs has already been outlined, but in this case they failed to even observe this phenomenon in Vero E6 cell cultures. Instead, they tried another method in order to, "test the pathogenicity of the ZC45 agent." This consisted of taking 20 μl the ground-up bat intestinal tissue and injecting it directly into the brains of 3-day old BALB/c rats. (By weight it would be the equivalent of injecting several hundred millilitres of material into a human brain.[115]) The nonsense of injecting such biological tissue directly into the brains of inbred, compromised neonatal animals shouldn't need any further explanation. As is typical in virology experiments, there was no control group where similar biological material, said not to contain the virus, was injected directly into the brains of other baby rats. They reported that "suspected viral particles" were seen in some of the rat brains but at no point did they demonstrate the composition or biological function of such observed "suspected viral particles" in their slides. Additionally,

[114] Dan Hu, et al. "Genomic characterization and infectivity of a novel SARS-like coronavirus in Chinese bats", *Emerging microbes & infections,* 12 Sep 2018: https://doi.org/10.1038/s41426-018-0155-5

[115] Western Australian Government - Animal Resource Centre, "Rat and Mice Weights": https://www.arc.wa.gov.au/?page_id=125

"infection" was declared on the basis of positive RT-PCR tests that detected the same RNA sequences in the baby rats at the time of their sacrifice as had been injected into them recently — obviously not something that required the existence of a virus.

So without physically isolating any alleged viral particles they proceeded to homogenise, centrifuge and filter the intestinal samples before declaring, "the viral RNA was extracted with a Viral RNA Mini Kit (Qiagen, Hilden, Germany) according to the manufacturer's recommendations." (See page 71 for an explanation of why it is not possible for kits of this type to selectively extract RNA on the basis of its provenance, regardless of whether viruses exist or not.) A reverse transcription step then took place before PCR amplification of their brew. They claimed to sequence the full genome of [SL-CoV]ZC45 through 19 degenerated PCR primer pairs, "designed by multiple alignment of available SARS-CoV and bat SL-CoV sequences deposited in GenBank." In other words, their declaration of discovering a viral genome was based not on direct evidence of a virus but on detection of sequences of unestablished provenance aligned to yet more fictional 'virus' templates. It was not disclosed how much PCR amplification took place at this step but the "RT-PCR screening" step involved a first round of 40 cycles, followed by a second round of 30 cycles. Such ridiculous amplification would result in artefact, meaning the target sequences are "found" simply as a result of the process itself rather than necessarily being physically present in the samples.

Of note, the bat virus story has been in play since the 2003 SARS "outbreak" and apparently after thousands of years, the human race is now under constant threat from viruses percolating in Chinese bat caves. In 2005, the EcoHealth Alliance president, Dr Peter Daszak, co-authored a paper that appeared in *Science* titled, "Bats Are Natural Reservoirs of SARS-Like Coronaviruses."[116] In this study, Daszak and co. couldn't find any

---

[116] Wendong Li, et al., "Bats Are Natural Reservoirs of SARS-Like Coronaviruses", *Science*, 29 Sep 2005: https://doi.org/10.1126/science.1118391

'coronaviruses' in their selection of bats through the usual fraudulent technique of observing *in vitro* CPEs, stating that, "no virus has been isolated from fecal swabs of PCR-positive samples using Vero E6 cells." However, they were happy to declare they had evidence of such viruses through their nonsensically high (35-45) cycle PCR products obtained from crude bat samples. These were claimed to be 'viral sequences' because within virology's circular reasoning they 'found' the very 'viral' sequences that their PCR protocol was designed to detect. They duly warned the world that, "genetic diversity exists among zoonotic viruses in bats increasing the possibility of variants crossing the species barrier and causing outbreaks of disease in human populations." Unfortunately, this zoonotic folklore has spread from the virology literature into the imagination of the public. Daszak is a keen promoter and benefactor of the bat virus story and in 2015 advised his colleagues that in order to keep the revenue coming in, they would need to, "increase public understanding of the need for MCMs [medical countermeasures] such as a pan-influenza or pan-coronavirus vaccine."[117]

In any case, a branch of one of the imaginary coronavirus template trails leads back to one of the original claims made regarding the SARS-CoV genome, alleged to be the cause of the first SARS "outbreak." In April 2003, Yijun Ruan et al. submitted to GenBank their, "SARS coronavirus Sin2500, complete genome," which became accession number AY283794.1.[118] However, this genome was invented not by directly sequencing alleged viral particles of course but by sequencing the RNA in a Vero cell culture experiment through, "both shot-gun and specific priming approaches," with alignment to, "the mouse hepatitis virus

---

117 "Developing MCMs for Coronaviruses", in Rapid Medical Countermeasure Response to Infectious Diseases: Enabling Sustainable Capabilities Through Ongoing Public- and Private-Sector Partnerships: Workshop Summary, Washington DC: National Academies Press, 12 Feb 2016: https://www.ncbi.nlm.nih.gov/books/NBK349040/

118 GenBank, "SARS coronavirus Sin2500, complete genome - AY283794.1", 27 Apr 2003: https://www.ncbi.nlm.nih.gov/nuccore/30468042

genome sequence (NC_001846) as a backbone."[119] The NC_001846.1 genome was invented in turn in 1997 and was claimed to be derived from a virus that was, "obtained originally from Dr. Lawrence Sturman," and sequenced, "using as templates, cytoplasmic RNA extracted from L2 cell monolayers infected with wild type MHV-A59, C12, C3, C5, C8, B11, or B12."[120] The assertion that they started with a virus appears to be based on Dr Sturman's assurance that the sample he provided contained such a thing.

It should be clear at this point that each coronavirus genome has been templated against other so-called genomes without the virologists demonstrating that *any* of the sequences come from a virus. It is thus instructive to go back to the purported first ever complete coronavirus genome to be published, which was the 'Avian Infectious Bronchitis Virus' (IBV) by Boursnell et al. in 1987,[121] and subsequently used by others as one of the original templates. They did not sequence any postulated viral particles directly but used, "seventeen cDNA clones covering the 3'-most 27,569 kb of the genome," noting that the clones, "have been derived from RNA isolated from gradient-purified virus of the Beaudette strain (Beaudette & Hudson, 1937; Brown & Boursnell, 1984)." The cited Brown & Boursnell paper states, "the preparation of cDNA clones has been previously described (Brown and Boursnell, 1984)."[122] This subsequent citation is their publication titled, "Avian infectious bronchitis

---

119 Yijun Ruan, et al., "Comparative full-length genome sequence analysis of 14 SARS coronavirus isolates and common mutations associated with putative origins of infection", *Lancet*, 24 May 2003: https://www.ncbi.nlm.nih.gov/pmc/articles/PMC7140172/

120 Isabelle Leparc-Goffart, et al., "Altered Pathogenesis of a Mutant of the Murine Coronavirus MHV-A59 Is Associated with a Q159L Amino Acid Substitution in the Spike Protein", *Virology*, 8 Dec 1997: https://doi.org/10.1006/viro.1997.8877

121 Michael Boursnell, et al., "Completion of the Sequence of the Genome of the Coronavirus Avian Infectious Bronchitis Virus", *J gen Virol*, 1 Jan 1987: https://doi.org/10.1099/0022-1317-68-1-57

122 T.D.K. Brown & Michael Boursnell, "Sequencing of coronavirus IBV genomic RNA: a 195base open reading frame encoded by mRNA B", *Gene*, Jul-Aug 1984: https://doi.org/10.1016/0378-1119(84)90169-0

virus genomic RNA contains sequence homologies at the intergenic boundaries".[123] In this paper they claim that the, "IBV strain Beaudette was grown in 11-day-old embryonated eggs. Virions were isolated from allantoic fluid and purified by isopycnic[124] centrifugation on sucrose gradients." However, no evidence was provided in any of these papers that they: (a) had purified anything, let alone "virions", in the form of confirmatory electron micrographs, or (b) performed valid control experiments. All we can see is that they *assumed* viruses were present in their culture mixture and after centrifugation claimed the detected RNA sequences were from these imagined viruses.

The original claim that they were dealing with a virus (IBV) dates back to the 1930s and was based on the same flawed conclusions drawn from the methodology employed in the 1911 Rous sarcoma "virus" experiments (see page 25). In the case of IBV, material was taken from diseased chickens, passed through Berkefeld bacterial filters and then introduced into the respiratory tracts of other chickens.[125] On the basis that this could also make the recipient birds sick, it was declared that, "these results demonstrate the disease is caused by a filterable virus." However, at no time has any experiment demonstrated that an infectious particle is responsible for the toxic effects. In short, the subsequent "coronavirus" phylogenetic trees that have been created since the 1980s are not evidence of "evolving viruses," they are evidence of a multi-level marketing scheme that has no established physical product.

---

[123] T.D.K. Brown & Michael Boursnell "Avian infectious bronchitis virus genomic RNA contains sequence homologies at the intergenic boundaries", *Virus Research*, Jan 1984: https://doi.org/10.1016/0168-1702(84)90031-5

[124] Isopycnic centrifugation separates particles by density cf. rate zonal centrifugation separates particles by size: https://www.differencebetween.com/difference-between-rate-zonal-and-isopycnic-centrifugation/

[125] J. R Beach & O. W. Schalm, "A Filterable Virus, Distinct from that of Laryngotracheitis, the Cause of a Respiratory Disease of Chicks", *Poultry Science*, May 1936: https://doi.org/10.3382/ps.0150199

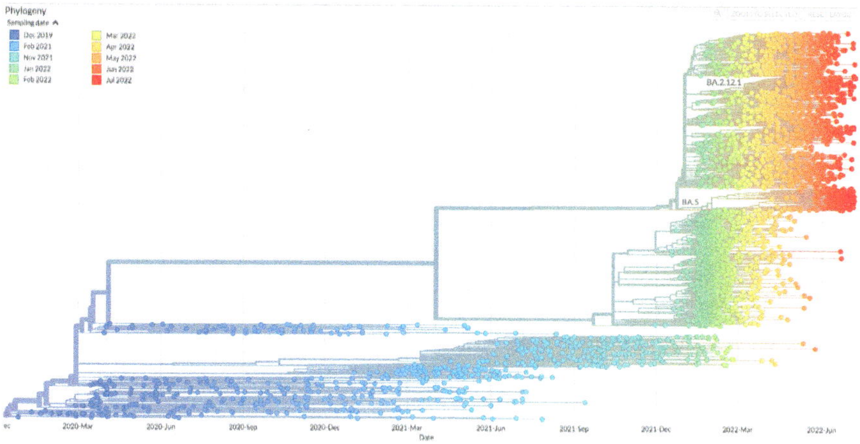

Figure 5. The SARS-CoV-2 phylogenetic tree on GISAID.org, as at 15 July 2022. The first "genome" from December 2019 (Fan Wu et al.) was never shown to come from a virus but through virology's circular reasoning similar sequences found in other places are proffered as evidence of an evolving "virus." However, the uncontrolled methodologies being utilised render it a fictional *in silico* family tree. Detecting, or purporting to detect selected genetic sequences in the environment does not confirm the existence of a virus given that the provenance of the sequences have not been established or have been misattributed. The same applies to detected proteins.

The danger to humanity is that the putative coronavirus genomes that have been templated out of the virologists' speculations are now used as templates to create and inject products into hapless recipients who were conned and gulled into believing that virology's latest invention was real. That is, virology's fictional genomic inventions have been relied upon to create wholly unnecessary medical and political interventions. The dangerous and highly experimental mRNA and nanolipid biotechnology has killed more people than all other vaccines combined over the last 30 years, and we have only just begun counting.[126]

[126] https://vaersanalysis.info/ (accessed 25 June 2022).

THE CDC'S CLAIM ON SARS-COV-2

With now familiar tardiness, the CDC took eight months to respond to a Freedom of Information request surrounding their claims of "isolating SARS-CoV-2" in their June 2020 *Emerging Infectious Diseases* publication, "Severe Acute Respiratory Syndrome Coronavirus 2 from Patient with Coronavirus Disease, United States," by Jennifer Harcourt et al.[127] The questions that were put to the CDC from my colleague were simple and included the following: "Did the scientist for this paper use control groups? If so, did the control groups use the same formulations of cell culture mixtures as the experimental groups *sans* the sample containing the alleged viruses?...In summary, if control groups were used, please list details of the control groups."[128] Instead of asking Jennifer Harcourt or one of her team to answer this simple request, on 29 March 2022, the CDC responded that they had, "located 37 pages of responsive records and one excel spreadsheet," allegedly pursuant to the material requested.[129] In summary, the CDC's "responsive records" included the following:[130]

1. Internal CDC emails sharing images such as Figure 6 below purporting to show, "scope pics of potential 2019 N-CoV from the 1st US case." CDC research microbiologists Azaibi Tamin hoped, "some of these 7 lysates show CPE are caused by the 2019 N-CoV," while Stephen Lindstrom commented they were, "very nice unhappy cells." The Respiratory virus immunology team lead, Natalie Thornburg then

---

[127] Jennifer Harcourt, et al., "Severe Acute Respiratory Syndrome Coronavirus 2 from Patient with Coronavirus Disease, United States", *Emerging Infectious Diseases*, June 2020: https://wwwnc.cdc.gov/eid/article/26/6/20-0516_article

[128] By email to FOIA Requests (CDC), "FOIA: Control Group Information requested for Severe Acute Respiratory Syndrome Coronavirus 2 from Patient with Coronavirus Disease, United States", 1 Aug 2021.

[129] Letter from Roger Andoh, CDC/ATSDR FOIA Officer, "#21-01704-FOIA", 29 Mar 2022: https://www.fluoridefreepeel.ca/wp-content/uploads/2022/05/CDC-Harcourt-mock-infected-MS-PACKAGE-redacted.pdf

[130] Ibid: 37-page PDF document from Roger Andoh, CDC/ATSDR FOIA Officer, "USA CDC - Controls - Responsive Records.pdf", 29 Mar 2022.

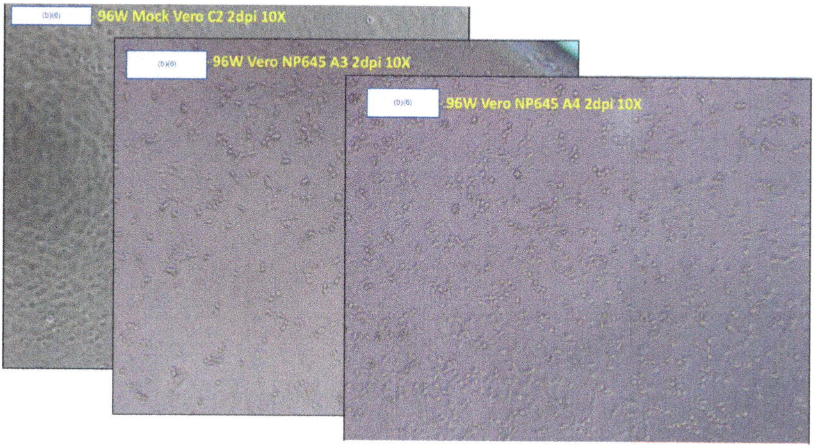

Figure 6. In their 29 March 2022 FOIA response, the details of the "mock" experiment slide were not provided by the CDC, despite being specifically requested. The other slides are supposedly evidence of the cytopathic effects (and thus *implied* existence) of SARS-CoV-2.

asked if they, "could send the original JPEG or TIFF files for your CPE images? I want to start working on a publication quality figure."

2. GenBank accession numbers MT020880 and MT020881, which were listed in the Harcourt et al./CDC publication and already publicly available.
3. The Na Zhu et al. *New England Journal of Medicine* paper, "A Novel Coronavirus from Patients with Pneumonia in China, 2019,"[131] which according to CDC electron microscopist Cynthia Goldsmith, "has 2 very nice EM images in Figure 3, one from 'human airway epithelial'." We dealt with the follies of this paper in *The COVID-19 Fraud & War on Humanity*, with Na Zhu et al. also being guilty of uncontrolled tissue culture breakdown experiments in which they christened electron micrographs of extracellular vesicles of unproven composition and

---

[131] Na Zhu et al., "A Novel Coronavirus from Patients with Pneumonia in China, 2019", *New England Journal of Medicine*, 382 (20 Feb 2020, first published 24 Jan 20, updated 29 Jan 2020), 728: https://pubmed.ncbi.nlm.nih.gov/31978945/

biological function "2019-nCoV".[132] (One of the paper's co-authors Wenjie Tan said to Torsten Engelbrecht on 18 March 2020 that they had, "an image of sedimented virus particles, not purified ones."[133] Thus, the claim that they are "virus particles" is simply an assertion, as there is no part of the paper that demonstrated the composition or biological function of these imaged vesicles.)

4. A spreadsheet with non-informative PCR cycle threshold results for "4 viruses" that were submitted to the CDC's Respiratory Viruses Diagnostic Laboratory.
5. A page starting with, "for administrative convenience and to fully respond to your request, program staff have provided the following information below with corresponding web links," which provided absolutely no information related to how the CDC's "viral isolation" experiments were suitably controlled.

On 23 December 2021, Christine Massey also submitted a request to the CDC seeking full details of the Harcourt et al. "mock infected" experiment including, "the quantity of material from uninfected nasopharyngeal and oropharyngeal swab specimens that was added to the cell culture control group."[134] The CDC eventually responded to Massey's request on 10 May 2022 with 36 pages of similarly unhelpful information and the excuse that:

> *In regards to certain portions of your request, a search of our records failed to reveal any documents pertaining to your request. These portions relate to your request for specific "... Cell Culture - Experimental Group Details:" and "Cell Culture - 'Mock-infected'/Control Group Details:" and "'Whole*

---

132 Mark Bailey & John Bevan-Smith, "The COVID-19 Fraud & War on Humanity", 11 Nov 2021: https://drsambailey.com/covid-19/the-covid-19-fraud-war-on-humanity/

133 Torsten Engelbrecht & Konstantin Demeter, "COVID19 PCR Tests are Scientifically Meaningless", *off-Guardian*, 27 Jun 2020: https://off-guardian.org/2020/06/27/covid19-pcr-tests-are-scientifically-meaningless/

134 Christine Massey, by email to CDC, "FOIA request to CDC: Harcourt et al. 'SARS-COV2 isolation' paper - unpublished details", 23 Dec 2021: https://www.fluoridefreepeel.ca/wp-content/uploads/2022/05/CDC-Harcourt-mock-infected-CM-PACKAGE-redacted.pdf

> *Genome' Sequencing - Purity and Control Details:" Your request was sent to the National Center for Immunization and Respiratory Diseases (NCIRD) for search. They responded that certain details in your request were not available as records controlled or maintained by CDC.*[135]

In other words, the CDC appear completely ignorant to the fact that they are not following the scientific method or they have realised that the game is up and are engaging in disingenuous responses. Either way, they cannot be taken seriously as a source of reliable scientific information if they are also promoting uncontrolled experiments as proof of viruses.

THE DISCLOSURES OF PENG ZHOU ET AL.

There have been occasions when investigators have provided responses regarding their methodologies where, intentionally or not, they are surprisingly candid about their unscientific experiments. On 3 February 2020, Peng Zhou et al. published their paper, "A pneumonia outbreak associated with a new coronavirus of probable bat origin," in *Nature,* claiming, "the identification and characterization of a new coronavirus (2019-nCoV)."[136] In their "isolation" experiment the authors produced images showing apparent CPEs in the alleged "2019-nCoV-infected" Vero E6 cells but no CPEs in the "mock-infected cells,"[137] the latter purported to be a "control." But what was the nature of this apparent control experiment? The details were not provided in their published paper so they were contacted by one of my colleagues in August 2021 who

---

[135] Letter from Emerique Magyar, CDC/ATSDR FOIA Officer to Christine Massey, "#22-00578-FOIA", 10 May 2022: https://www.fluoridefreepeel.ca/wp-content/uploads/2022/05/CDC-Harcourt-mock-infected-CM-PACKAGE-redacted.pdf

[136] Peng Zhou, et al., "A pneumonia outbreak associated with a new coronavirus of probable bat origin", *Nature*, 579, 12 Mar 2020: https://www.nature.com/articles/s41586-020-2012-7

[137] Ibid. "Extended Data Fig. 6: Isolation and antigenic characterization of 2019-nCoV": https://www.nature.com/articles/s41586-020-2012-7/figures/9

extracted some startling admissions from one of the paper's co-authors, Xing-Lou Yang. Firstly, aside from the fact that there were no positive control experiments (i.e. with comparable human samples minus the alleged virus), Yang stated they doubled the dose of penicillin and streptomycin in the experimental group.[138] When asked why this variable was altered, the response was, "the intention of Anti-Anti [the two antibiotics] is to prevent contamination from bacteria or fungi during virus isolation, so 1% or 2% concentration did not affect the cell growth. 2% in 1st gen [generation] was just to prevent contamination from samples."[139]

My colleague suggested that they should run the "control" experiment again with the higher dose antibiotics to ensure that this was not one of the factors inducing CPEs in the kidney cell line. Yang subsequently provided the evasive response, "if you could make sure that you could prevent contamination from bac [bacteria] or fungi, you do not need to use the Anti-Anti,"[140] seemingly ignoring the crucial point that it could be the additional antibiotics themselves that were toxic to the cells (particularly as streptomycin is known to be nephrotoxic). At the least, they had altered other variables compared with their controls and had thus invalidated their results even further.

Another staggering revelation from the authors was that in their experimental group, only *one* out of 24 wells containing Vero E6 kidney cell cultures (and only *one* out of 24 wells containing Huh7 cell cultures) showed any evidence of CPEs.[141] So, what should be considered an experimental margin of error is the basis of one of the declarations of a claimed deadly new pathogen, described in an article that, as of July 2022,

---

[138] (Personal correspondence by email from Xing-Lou Yang, 5 Aug 2021.)

[139] Ibid.

[140] Ibid.

[141] Ibid.

Control Group Vero E6

- Cell Culture Plate: 24 wells
- Cell Lines: Vero E6
- DMEM: 0.5 ml per well
- FBS: 2%
- Anti-Anti: 1%
- Trypsin: None

Experimental Group Vero E6

- Cell Culture Plate: 24 wells
- Cell Lines: Vero E6
- DMEM: 0.5ml per well
- FBS: 2%
- Anti-Anti: 2%(1st gen), 1% (next gen)
- Trypsin: None

Figure 7. The Peng Zhou et al. study and their previously undisclosed methodology: double the antibiotics in the experimental group to see CPEs in only one out of 24 wells. It is declared this constitutes evidence of a new viral pathogen '2019-nCoV', later to be renamed SARS-CoV-2.

has been accessed 1.34 million times and cited over 10 thousand times.[142] Do the other authors who are citing this paper realise the gossamer of "evidence" this house of cards called COVID-19 is built upon? Perhaps they would not be perturbed by such a revelation as biological experiments are being increasingly abandoned while *in silico* "genomes" are absurdly claimed to provide adequate evidence for the existence of viruses. In the case of Zhou et al., their computer simulation was proudly proclaimed to be, "96% identical at the whole-genome level to a bat coronavirus." They decided to template their new viral invention against this sequence, based on the nonsense that, "previous studies have shown that some bat SARSr-CoVs have the potential to infect humans."[143] Their software assembled what became GenBank accession numbers MN996527–MN996532 and this form of faux "evidence," which also lacks valid controls, has been documented in this essay.

---

[142] Article metrics, "A pneumonia outbreak associated with a new coronavirus of probable bat origin", *Nature*: https://www.nature.com/articles/s41586-020-2012-7/metrics (accessed 1 Apr 2022).

[143] Peng Zhou, et al., "A pneumonia outbreak associated with a new coronavirus of probable bat origin", *Nature*, 579, 12 Mar 2020: https://www.nature.com/articles/s41586-020-2012-7

MORE DECEPTION FROM WUHAN?

In early 2022, a mathematician working with Dr Stefan Lanka released an analysis of the associated sequence data produced by Fan Wu et al.[144] Startlingly, it was concluded that:

> *a repeat of the de novo assembly with Megahit (v.1.2.9) showed that the published results could not be reproduced. We may have detected (ribosomal) ribonucleic acids of human origin, contrary to what was reported [by Fan Wu et al.]...Evidence is lacking that only viral nucleic acids were used to construct the claimed viral genome for SARS-CoV-2. Further, with respect to the construction of the claimed viral genome strand, no results of possible control experiments have been published. This is equally true for all other reference sequences considered in the present work. In the case of SARS-CoV-2, an obvious control would be that the claimed viral genome cannot be assembled from unsuspected RNA sources of human, or even other, origin.*

Aside from the fact that virology's current methodologies for finding viruses should be rejected, the lack of reproducibility of their own experiment instantly raises questions about the circumstances in which the original inventors of SARS-CoV-2 announced their new virus to the world. Indeed, this independent analysis only obtained 28,459 contigs, significantly less than the number (384,096) described by Fan Wu et al. Additionally, the longest contig independently obtained was 29,802 nucleotides, which was 672 nucleotides shorter than Fan Wu's, meaning that, "the published sequence data cannot be the original reads used for assembly."

---

[144]"Strukturelle Analyse von Sequenzdaten in der Virologie · tabellen und Abbildungen", *WiSSeNSCHAFFtPLUS magazin*, Jan 2022. English version: https://brandfolder.com/s/3z266k74ppmnwkvfrxs6jjc

The mathematician's analysis also concluded that:

> *Alignment with the nucleotide database on 05/12/2021 showed a high match (98.85%) with "Homo sapiens RNA, 45S preribosomal N4 (RNA45SN4), ribosomal RNA" (GenBank: NR_146117.1, dated 04/07/2020). This observation contradicts the claim in [1] that ribosomal RNA depletion was performed and human sequence reads were filtered using the human reference genome (human release 32, GRCh38.p13). Of particular note here is the fact that the sequence NR_146117.1 was not published until after the publication of the SRR10971381 sequence library considered here. This observation emphasizes the difficulty of determining a priori the exact origin of the individual nucleic acid fragments used to construct claimed viral genome sequences.*

In any case, the problems didn't end there. The coverage distribution for some of the contigs was extremely inhomogeneous and given the high error rate, it raised the question of whether some of the sequences were simply those generated by the PCR amplification conditions themselves. Again, it is an anti-scientific method as appropriate control experiments (with similar human-derived samples) are not performed to examine these possibilities. The independent analysis revealed that Fan Wu et al. could have found better *in silico* consensus matches for 'HIV' and 'Hepatitis D virus' than "a new coronavirus" in their 41-year-old man from Wuhan, who presented with pneumonia as one of the first claimed COVID-19 cases. If the virologists want to find a virus, it all depends on how they design their protocols and what they ask the computer to look for — and how would these fortune tellers know what to look for?

PROFESSOR STEPHEN BUSTIN'S PRIMING OF A PCR PANDEMIC

Scientists have a tendency to assume that everything outside of their domain of interest is true and that they can just rely on it.

— David Crowe following his interview of Stephen Bustin in April 2020.[145]

To sustain the illusion of the COVID-19 'pandemic', cases were required. These were provided by the world's largest ever human 'testing' programme involving billions of PCR kits distributed around the world. It remains unclear to us as to why Stephen Bustin, who is a, "world-renowned expert on quantitative PCR, and his research focuses on translating molecular techniques into practical, robust and reliable tools for clinical and diagnostic use,"[146] failed to decisively point out the inappropriate use of the PCR process. Bustin was the lead author for the 2009 publication, "The MIQE Guidelines: Minimum Information for Publication of Quantitative Real-Time PCR Experiments,"[147] in which the key conceptual considerations for real-time PCR experiments were outlined as follows:

1. *2.1* ***Analytical sensitivity*** *refers to the minimum number of copies in a sample that can be measured accurately with an assay, whereas* ***clinical sensitivity*** *is the percentage of individuals with a given disorder whom the assay identifies as positive for that condition…*

---

145 *The Infectious Myth* with David Crowe - "Simplifying RT-PCR", 21 Apr 2020: https://infectiousmyth.podbean.com/e/the-infectious-myth-simplifying-rt-pcr/

146 https://aru.ac.uk/people/stephen-bustin

147 Stephen Bustin, et al., "The MIQE Guidelines: Minimum Information for Publication of Quantitative Real-Time PCR Experiments", *Clinical Chemistry*, 1 Apr 2009: https://doi.org/10.1373/clinchem.2008.112797

2. *2.2 **Analytical specificity** refers to the qPCR assay detecting the appropriate target sequence rather than other, nonspecific targets also present in a sample. **Diagnostic specificity** is the percentage of individuals without a given condition whom the assay identifies as negative for that condition.*

If Bustin remained true to the science then he should have called a halt to the PCR pandemic in January 2020 when the Corman-Drosten PCR protocols were published.[148] The word 'specificity' appears only once in the Corman-Drosten paper and it had nothing to do with diagnosing a clinical condition, let alone a viral infection. There was no "detection of 2019-nCoV" as the paper claimed, all that was established was the analytical specificity of their assay to detect selected target sequences. It was an *in vitro* molecular reaction experiment with synthetic nucleic acid technology that does not require the existence of a virus. Further, there was no establishment of how the PCR result related to a clinical condition, i.e. the COVID-19 PCR kits were never shown to diagnose anything in a human subject. An invented disease based on a fictional virus.

Aside from the issue of specificity, it was not well publicised that the world-expert on PCR said to David Crowe in April 2020 that, (even on virology's own terms,) calling a coronavirus PCR result "positive" at 36-37 cycles, as was happening around the world was, "absolute nonsense. It makes no sense whatsoever."[149] However, the PCR fraud was even more apparent when Eric Coppolino interviewed Bustin on *Planet Waves FM* in February 2021.[150] Coppolino's intention was to find out more details about

---

[148] Victor Corman, et al., "Detection of 2019 novel coronavirus (2019-nCoV) by real-time RT-PCR", *EuroSurveillance*, 23 Jan 2020: https://doi.org/10.2807/1560-7917.ES.2020.25.3.2000045.

[149] *The Infectious Myth* with David Crowe, "Stephen Bustin on Challenges with RT-PCR", 14 Apr 2020: https://infectiousmyth.podbean.com/e/the-infectious-myth-stephen-bustin-on-challenges-with-rt-pcr/

[150] *Planet Waves FM* with Eric F. Coppolino, "Interview with Dr. Stephen Bustin", 1 Feb 2021: https://planetwaves.net/planet-waves-fm-interview-with-dr-stephen-bustin/

the problematic reverse transcription (RT) step of the RT-PCR process but he was stunned after the interview to realise that what he thought was a sometimes inaccurate test was completely fraudulent.[151] Bustin appeared uncomfortable when Coppolino pointed out that all positive PCR results were being called a, "confirmed case of infection," even if they had no symptoms.[152] Instead of admitting that the diagnostic specificity of the PCR kits had never been established, Bustin offered peripheral explanations such as claiming that, "ICUs are overrun at the moment."

He further defended the PCR protocols in use with the assertion that, "this pneumonia was being caused by this virus. And this virus started popping up where more and more people were coming down with the same symptoms. And these primers were detecting that virus." When Coppolino pushed him on the lack of virus isolation to be able to make these claims, Bustin responded that, "the way the sequence was established by taking the samples from the original patient, growing up something and then sequencing it and then disassembling the sequence and what came out of that was the SARS virus." Unfortunately, Bustin lent support to virology's misuse of the word 'isolation' and the loose terminology involved in detecting a "virus." The crucial issue is that it doesn't matter how well designed any primers are — if the provenance or significance of the genetic sequences being amplified through the PCR are unknown, then nothing more can be concluded by their mere presence. Bustin can reassure the world about the potentially very high analytical performance of a PCR protocol but the establishment of its diagnostic performance is where the rubber meets the road. Even if SARS-CoV-2 had been shown to physically exist and the PCR was accepted as a valid diagnostic tool, Bustin would have to admit that none of the PCR assays have been developed as his *MIQE Guidelines* specify and none qualify as being clinically-validated.

---

151 (Personal correspondence from Eric Coppolino.)

152 *Planet Waves FM* with Eric F. Coppolino, "Interview with Dr. Stephen Bustin", 1 Feb 2021: https://planetwaves.net/planet-waves-fm-interview-with-dr-stephen-bustin/

It was a surprise during the same interview that he denied any prior knowledge of the false pertussis outbreak in Dartmouth-Hitchcock, New Hampshire in 2006 when the PCR kit that was rolled out resulted in a 100% false positive rate.[153] Bustin claimed to have learned about it for the first time just days before the interview, some 15 years after the fact, when he read about it on Coppolino's website, from an article provided for the purposes of the interview. Yet the incident was well known and received coverage in *The New York Times*, with comments from many public health and diagnostic test professionals.[154] By 2006, Bustin was a Professor of Molecular Biology and it is a small wonder that the PCR specialist had not had any enquiries from medical colleagues in 2006 when the incident happened. Indeed, at the time there were very few PCR experts in existence to contact and it was an early indication of how the PCR could be catastrophically misused as a clinical diagnostic tool. If that wasn't bad enough, it related to an incident where the purportedly causal microbe (the bacterium *Bordetella pertussis*) is something that can be physically isolated and its genetic sequences confirmed for the PCR to be calibrated against. In contrast, the SARS-CoV-2 PCR protocols are simply calibrated to genetic fragments of unknown origin. When Coppolino pressed him on this point Bustin responded, "well, you know, this is a standard way of doing this so I really can't comment any further on that, except that to me that's perfectly acceptable and that's the way to do it."[155]

By the time Bustin was interviewed by Coppolino he had already co-authored and submitted a paper titled, "COVID-19 and Diagnostic Testing for SARS-CoV-2 by RT-qPCR—Facts and Fallacies" that was published later

---

153 CDC, "Outbreaks of Respiratory Illness Mistakenly Attributed to Pertussis - New Hampshire, Massachusetts, and Tennessee, 2004-2006", *Morbidity and Mortality Weekly Report*, 24 Aug 2007: https://www.cdc.gov/mmwr/preview/mmwrhtml/mm5633a1.htm

154 Gina Kolata, "Faith in Quick Test Leads to Epidemic That Wasn't", *The New York Times*, 22 Jan 2007: https://www.nytimes.com/2007/01/22/health/22whoop.html

155 *Planet Waves FM* with Eric F. Coppolino, "Interview with Dr. Stephen Bustin", 1 Feb 2021: https://planetwaves.net/planet-waves-fm-interview-with-dr-stephen-bustin/

in February 2021.[156] In this paper, Bustin and co stated that, "[the Corman-Drosten] assay worked and was specific and demonstrated astounding sagacity and selflessness by the scientists involved, as well as the remarkable speed with which PCR-based tests can be developed and put into practice." Ignoring the fawning praise, the obvious question remains, is specific for what? Were Bustin and co implying that the PCR tests are specific for (a) short targeted RNA sequences, (b) a coronavirus known as SARS-CoV-2, or (c) the WHO-invented disease known as COVID-19? The Corman-Drosten paper only established the analytical specificity for amplifying some selected RNA sequences, it had nothing to do with the establishment of a virus or diagnosing a disease. The developer of the *MIQE Guidelines* surely knows that of the three, only the first was scientifically established and nothing was, or has been, validated for clinical application. And yet his paper goes on to make the ridiculous *non sequitur* that, "PCR testing is highly suitable for large scale testing, as demonstrated daily by the millions of tests carried out to date." Has Bustin forgotten that the 'tests' are simply a molecular amplification tool? As the inventor of the PCR, Dr Kary Mullis warned in 1993, "I don't think you can misuse PCR, no, the results, the interpretation of it [is misused]."[157]

The PCR simply amplifies selected genetic sequences and the molecular reaction itself has no capacity to determine their provenance or the relevance of their presence. If a particular PCR protocol is performed correctly and has a known 100% analytical sensitivity and specificity, a positive result can be said to have done nothing more than confirmed the presence of a target sequence. However, if claims are being made that the PCR is a diagnostic tool, it should be obvious that clinical validation studies would need to be performed before the test was introduced into clinical

---

156 Stephen Bustin, et al., "COVID-19 and Diagnostic Testing for SARS-CoV-2 by RT-qPCR—Facts and Fallacies", *Int. J. Mol. Sci.*, 28 Feb 2021: https://doi.org/10.3390/ijms22052459

157 David James, "PCR Inventor: 'It doesn't tell you that you are sick'", *off-Guardian*, 5 Oct 2020: https://off-guardian.org/2020/10/05/pcr-inventor-it-doesnt-tell-you-that-you-are-sick/

practice. The Corman-Drosten paper skipped this step and the WHO accepted the fraud by placing versions of the PCR protocol on their website on the 13th and then 17th of January, 2020, before the paper had even been published.[158] After that the PCR was simply used via circular reasoning to make claims about diagnosing "infections" in people.

The next phase in the early stages of the alleged pandemic involved "experts" such as Australian Infectious Diseases Specialist, Associate Professor Sanjaya Senanayake promulgating unfounded claims about the accuracy of the tests to the public. In an interview on the 26th of April, 2020 he stated that with regard to COVID-19 testing, "there's no real gold standard to compare this to...for COVID-19 we don't have a gold standard test so so the current tests we are using, the PCR tests...they're our gold standard, but trying to work around that, we think that it's probably picking up around 70% of cases."[159] Senanayake implied that if you don't have a gold standard you can just assume that a new PCR test can validate itself. However, this goes against all scholarship regarding test validation. It is unclear through this departure from the established tenets of validation logic how he calculated that it worked "about 70%" of the time, not to mention the mental gymnastics involved in a "gold standard" that detects itself only 70% of the time. It would be agreed with his inadvertent admission that, "there's no real gold standard" in COVID-19 testing because the real gold standard is something that doesn't exist — that being the physical isolation and proof of a viral particle.

The WHO were not concerned by the lack of a gold standard or evidence of a virus and cemented the PCR fraud by stating that a COVID-19 case was, "a person with laboratory [in 2020, typically PCR] confirmation of

---

[158] Victor Corman, et al., "Diagnostic detection of 2019-nCoV by real-time RT-PCR", WHO, 17 Jan 2020: https://www.who.int/docs/default-source/coronaviruse/protocol-v2-1.pdf?sfvrsn=a9ef618c_2

[159] Sanjaya Senanayake being interviewed by Jeremy Fernandez on *The Virus*, ABC News, 26 Apr 2020: https://iview.abc.net.au/show/virus/series/0/video/NC2032H003S00

COVID-19 infection, irrespective of clinical signs and symptoms."[160] In this one sentence, they proclaim that the clinically unvalidated PCR tests have 100% diagnostic specificity, and nonsensically twist the meaning of the word "infection" to include individuals who have no signs or symptoms. The etymology of the word 'infection' provides a derivation from the Latin *inficere*, meaning 'to stain'. Mosby's Medical Dictionary 2009 states the definition of infection to be, "(1) the invasion of the body by pathogenic microorganisms that reproduce and multiply, causing disease by local cellular injury, secretion of a toxin, or antigen-antibody reaction in the host, and (2) a disease caused by the invasion of the body by pathogenic microorganisms."[161]

While the author makes no pronouncement as to any microbes being pathogenic, the established meaning of 'infection' relates to a disease state — otherwise a term such as 'commensalism'[162] should be used. The WHO invented an absurd new definition of 'pandemic'[163] and are now subverting the definition of infection — one that disconnects it from the concept of disease through the sole use of PCR results. Kary Mullis couldn't have put it any simpler when he said the PCR is, "just a process that's used to make a whole lot of something out of something."[164] Unfortunately, on more than one occasion in the COVID-19 era, influential figures such as Bustin and Senanayake have supported the virologists use

---

160 WHO, "WHO COVID-19: Case Definitions", 7 Aug 2020: https://www.who.int/publications/i/item/WHO-2019-nCoV-Surveillance_Case_Definition-2020.1

161 Mosby's Medical Dictionary - 8th edition, 2009, Elsevier.

162 The Merriam-Webster Dictionary defines commensalism as "a relation between two kinds of organisms in which one obtains food or other benefits from the other without damaging or benefiting it": https://www.merriam-webster.com/dictionary/commensalism (accessed 14 May 2022).

163 Ron Law, "WHO and the pandemic flu 'conspiracies'", Rapid response, 6 Jun 2010: https://www.bmj.com/rapid-response/2011/11/02/who-changed-definition-influenza-pandemic

164 David James, "PCR Inventor: 'It doesn't tell you that you are sick'", *off-Guardian*, 5 Oct 2020: https://off-guardian.org/2020/10/05/pcr-inventor-it-doesnt-tell-you-that-you-are-sick/.

of a molecular manufacturing tool to make all sorts of unfounded claims, including both the unratified ability to diagnose a novel infection and the detection of an alleged virus.

Of note, a biased misinterpretation of the PCR appears to begin before the amplification process has even started. For example, the Roche "High Pure Viral RNA Kit," used to prepare samples for the PCR, states that it, "rapidly isolates viral RNA from mammalian plasma, serum, body fluids, and cell culture supernatants."[165] It is unclear from the supplied product information how the kit would separate alleged viral RNA from other RNA present in the sample.[166] The process includes a "poly(A) carrier RNA" binding additive step, but polyadenylated sequences are non-specific,[167] and the following buffering and centrifugation steps they describe would not be able to differentiate the provenance of the RNA either. Despite this, the "protocols" section proclaims that the end product is "purified viral RNA,"[168] so that anyone believing this unfounded claim thinks their subsequent positive RT-PCR result is evidence of a virus. The same can be said for Roche's "High Pure Viral Nucleic Acid Kit," used by teams such as Na Zhu's and Peng Zhou's in their claims to have discovered SARS-CoV-2 in patient specimens and cell culture experiments. Once again Roche make the spurious statement that the steps outlined in the "protocols" section would result in "purified viral nucleic acids."[169]

---

165 Roche, "High Pure Viral RNA Kit - Product No. 11858882001": https://lifescience.roche.com/en_au/products/high-pure-viral-rna-kit.html

166 Roche, "'High Pure Viral RNA Kit - Version: 20, Cat. No. 11 858 882 001' Instructions for Use", Oct 2020: https://pim-eservices.roche.com/LifeScience/Document/96aae49e-ad12-eb11-fe90-005056a772fd

167 Mary Edmonds, "A history of poly A sequences: from formation to factors to function", *Prog Nucleic Acid Res Mol Biol*, Vol 71, 2002: https://doi.org/10.1016/S0079-6603(02)71046-5

168 Roche, "'High Pure Viral RNA Kit - Version: 20, Cat. No. 11 858 882 001' Instructions for Use", Oct 2020: https://pim-eservices.roche.com/LifeScience/Document/96aae49e-ad12-eb11-fe90-005056a772fd

169 Roche, "'High Pure Viral Nucleic Acid Kit - Version: 20, Cat. No. 11 858 874 001' Instructions for Use", Oct 2020: https://pim-eservices.roche.com/LifeScience/Document/d927229f-ad12-eb11-0091-005056a71a5d

Incidentally, Bustin was asked specifically about Roche's claims when the following was put to him: "I assume the kit must be able to distinguish viral NAs [nucleic acids] from all the others. Do viral NAs have a chemically unique property?" He responded, "the extraction process is not specific for any particular nucleic acid but it can be specific for types of nucleic acid. Some kits can differentials [*sic*] extract *DNA or RNA*, but this means *any DNA and RNA* will be present in the extracted sample [my emphasis]... A small amount of the extracted material is then subjected to the PCR reaction. This is what provides the specificity."[170] In other words, Bustin did not attempt to provide an explanation for Roche's fraudulent claims, but obfuscated the issue by substituting the specificity of provenance of the nucleic acids with the specificity of the sequences being selected for the PCR. This amounts to a linguistic sleight of hand that helped allow a "virus" to appear out of thin air.

170 (Personal correspondence from Stephen Bustin to my colleague, 15 Oct 2021.)

PART THREE

"LITTLE MOUNTAIN DOG" — NAÏVE OR GASLIGHTING?

I would never have seen it if I hadn't believed it.

— Ashleigh Brilliant[171]

We are familiar with the allegation that it would be impossible for the majority of the medical and scientific community to all be knowingly complicit with virology's unscientific methodologies in the COVID-19 fraud. The author does not advance such a hypothesis, although it is wondered whether and for how long ignorance may be used as a defence? Indeed, that is why it was suggested earlier in this essay (in 'What Is Virology?') that, "the abandonment of the scientific method may be unnoticed or accidental by lower level participants." Freshly-minted virologists are trained to follow the methodologies of their seniors and are unlikely to get far with their chosen career, and of course funding, if they dispute the basis of their laboratory's work.

On 29 January 2020, an apparent Chinese virology scientist known as "Winjor Little Mountain Dog" posted a text titled, "Documenting the first experience of discovering a novel coronavirus."[172] It described the impassioned story of an insider determined to get the truth out regarding what happened in Wuhan over the preceding month and who really 'discovered' WH-Human 1 aka 'WH-01/2019', later to be renamed 'SARS-CoV-2'. To those of us aware of the deception that has taken place in the COVID-19 charade, the text is certainly suspicious as being part of a

---

171 https://www.ashleighbrilliant.com/

172 "记录一下首次发现新型冠状病毒的经历", 29 Jan 2020: https://freewechat.com/a/MzAxMjMyMDk0Ng==/2650112053/1/1580318101, One of the English translations: "Documenting the first experience of discovering a novel coronavirus": https://github.com/flodebarre/covid_origin_documents/blob/main/2020-01-30_LittleDog.md

gaslighting operation. Otherwise, the relative ease in deducing which laboratory the story originated from makes the author appear extremely naïve for an inhabitant of the communist Chinese state. However, the document will be presented as it is described; that is with the narrator believing they were discovering viruses in the following selected passages.

> *I just went to work on December 26, 2019. As usual, I will first browse the results of the automatic interpretation of mNGS pathogenic microorganisms for this day.*

Here the author described their laboratory performing metagenomic NGS on crude patient specimens as outlined in preceding sections of this essay. It set the theme for the author's text, which described 'viruses' in terms of genetic sequences that can be detected in the environment and assembled by computer software.

> *Unexpectedly, it was found that one sample reported a sensitive pathogen - SARS coronavirus, with dozens of sequences, and this sample has only such a meaningful pathogen.*

This is an incredible leap from various sequences that have been detected in a crude specimen to the report of a "pathogen," apparently on the basis that this can be established by a computer program. Not only that but the computer has found a "SARS coronavirus" so it is somehow known to be associated with the clinical condition 'severe acute respiratory syndrome'.

> *...this pathogen is most similar to Bat SARS like coronavirus, with an overall similarity of about 87%, and a similarity to SARS* [SARS-CoV-1] *of about 81%. The number of sequences in the alignment has increased from dozens to more than 500. In addition, 5 contigs have been assembled, which add up to more than 1200 bp. At this time, it can basically be confirmed*

> *that it is a coronavirus...In such an urgent situation, there is no time to research the literature, and there is not much data in hand...We further analyzed thousands of coronavirus genomes in a carpet-like manner, and evaluated them in terms of similarity, coverage, and even genome distribution, and finally found the two most similar genomes, bat-SL-CoVZC45 and bat-SL-CoVZXC21.*

And just like that, it is "confirmed" that the virus existed on the basis of comparing some new *in silico* assemblies with other *in silico* assemblies previously submitted to genetic databases. The author goes on to describe their next activity of phylogenetic tree analysis and building an evolutionary path for the latest addition to virology's fictional family tree. There is a complete absence of any appreciation of the fact that a virus must possess an actual physical existence as a discrete particle with specific biological characteristics, including the ability to infect hosts and *cause* disease. The author simply asserted that, "the analysis has basically confirmed that there is indeed a virus in the sample of this patient." Later in the text they sound some caution with regard to clinical pathogenicity but remain convinced of its existence by making the passing comment that, "whether the pneumonia was caused by this virus, we did not analyze it, nor could we analyze it. The detection of the virus does not mean that the pneumonia was caused by the virus."

> *...by December 30, I heard that there are quite a few patients with similar symptoms...What really made me nervous again was that a friend and businessman shared the sequence for us to analyze. I analyzed it, and it was indeed the same virus! The first thought in the subconscious is "this virus is contagious"!*

It is unclear whether the author knew that "similar symptoms" afflicting the patients described in Wuhan were all non-specific respiratory symptoms. To this day COVID-19 is not a legitimately-defined *clinical* condition, as the "confirmed" cases simply refer to the result of a molecular detection process.[173] Additionally, we have already dealt with the circular reasoning and self-referential process of inventing a 'virus genome' through virology's methodology and then claiming that detection of almost identical assemblies in other places is confirmation that "the same virus" has been found.[174]

> *The nervousness is that this unknown virus may be as terrifying as SARS; the excitement is that we detected and confirmed this pathogen early through mNGS technology, and quarantined the patient, and it may be possible to prevent and control the virus before it spreads widely, strangled in the cradle!...I also hope that after we have experienced this new coronavirus incident, the country's ability to handle major public health events has made great progress...As far as I know, we should have been the first to discover this virus, because it was after we reported the results that the disease control system began to intervene.*

It is up to the reader to decide whether the author truly believed that they were the first to discover SARS-CoV-2 and that public health experts have these abilities, or if this text was engineered and "leaked" as another part of the COVID-19 propaganda. There was never any virus to spread. The only thing that was spreading around the world, aside from fear, was the fictional WH-Human 1 'genome' and the PCR tests that were calibrated to its sequences. The 'pandemic' could have been stopped in its tracks by the

---

173 "WHO COVID-19 Case definitions: Updated in Public health surveillance for COVID-19 | COVID-19: Surveillance, case investigation and epidemiological protocol", 16 Dec 2020: https://www.who.int/publications/i/item/WHO-2019-nCoV-Surveillance_Case_Definition-2020.2 (The small footnote does state: "Surveillance case definitions should not be used as the sole basis for guiding clinical management.")

174 Mark Bailey & John Bevan-Smith, "The COVID-19 Fraud & War on Humanity", 11 Nov 2021: https://drsambailey.com/covid-19/the-covid-19-fraud-war-on-humanity/

rejection of these tests; instead ignorant public health "experts" bought into virology's anti-science and have been parties to the COVID-19 fraud since.

Little Mountain Dog purportedly wanted it to be known that their laboratory was, "the first to discover the virus," following the collection of their Wuhan sample on 24 December 2019, and the subsequent submission to the GISAID database on 11 January 2020 as accession ID 'EPI_ISL_402123'. Along with the *in silico* sequence from Fan Wu et al., EPI_ISL_402123 was used in the design of the PCR protocols by Christian Drosten's team (shown in Figure 8 below). However, as David Rasnick pointed out, "they never touched a virus at all." This provides an element of irony to the "lab leak" hypothesis; a narrative that appeared in the mainstream media as early February 2020.[175] The "virus" was certainly invented in a lab but it was a computer lab and the only entity that was intentionally leaked out was a computer simulation. The results of the simulation were sent around the world as digital code over the internet and the resulting PCR primers that were deployed in kits *en masse* created the "cases" for the COVID-19 fraud.

The Little Mountain Dog story continued when an editorial entitled, "As the pandemic exploded, a researcher saw the danger. China's leaders kept silent" appeared in *The Washington Post* on 22 April 2022.[176] They reported that Little Mountain Dog was based in a commercial laboratory 'Vision Medicals' in Guangzhou in southern China and, "her story points to a coverup with tragic consequences of historic proportion. A severe danger was concealed until it was too late." The editorial promoted all of the virological claims at face value and ironically stated that, "the episode

[175] "Chronology for Covid & SARS-CoV-2 PCR and Metagenomics": https://chironreturn.org/

[176] Editorial Board, "As the pandemic exploded, a researcher saw the danger. China's leaders kept silent", *The Washington Post*, 22 Apr 2022: https://www.washingtonpost.com/opinions/interactive/2022/china-researcher-covid-19-coverup/

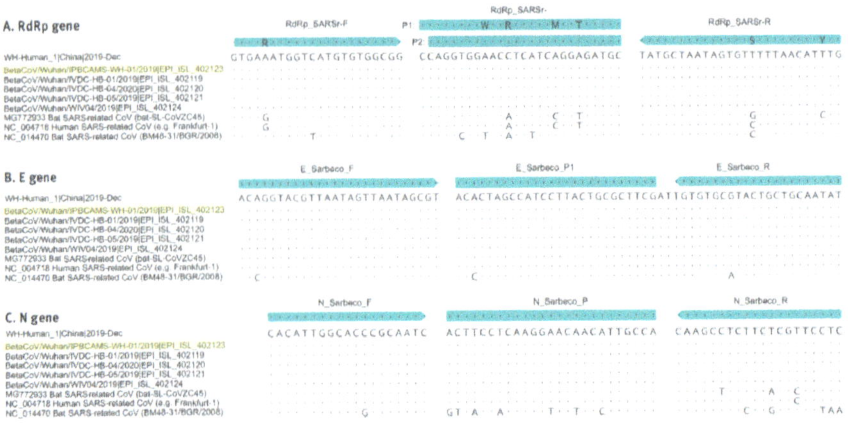

Figure 8. Little Mountain Dog's GISAID deposit 'EPI_ISL_402123'. It appeared alongside Fan Wu et al. deposit 'WH-Human_1|China|2019-Dec' for the Corman-Drosten RT-PCR protocol where it was stated, "the alignment [WH-Human_1|China|2019-Dec] was complemented by additional sequences released independently on GISAID." Source: "Detection of 2019 novel coronavirus (2019-nCoV) by real-time RT-PCR (Figure 2)."

serves to underscore once again why a serious investigation is needed to get to the bottom of how the pandemic began." A serious investigation of this topic demonstrates that at the bottom of this "pandemic" there is nothing more than nonsense, invented by the virologists and promulgated by outlets such as *The Washington Post*.

THE "LAB LEAK" DISTRACTION

> *You here assume smallpox to be a thing, an entity. This blunder is committed by nearly all the followers of the self-styled "regular school," and it will probably be a new idea to you to be told that neither smallpox nor any other disease is an entity, but is a condition.*
>
> — Dr Montague R. Leverson, 1909.[177]

[177] "English City of Leicester as Example of Benefits of Abolition of Vaccination", *Bridgeport Evening Farmer*, 21 Aug 1909.

On 19 May 2022, Jeffrey Sachs, the chair of the Lancet COVID-19 Commission, co-authored a paper with Neil Harrison entitled, "A call for an independent inquiry into the origin of the SARS-CoV-2 virus."[178] The publication opened with the following framing of the COVID-19 situation:

> *Since the identification of the* [sic] *SARS-CoV-2 in Wuhan, China, in January 2020, the origin of the virus has been a topic of intense scientific debate and public speculation. The two main hypotheses are that the virus emerged from human exposure to an infected animal ("zoonosis") or that it emerged in a research-related incident.*

However, alleging that there are "two main hypotheses" relies on the acceptance that, "the identification of SARS-CoV-2," means the particle has both a physical existence, and the specific biological properties required to fulfil the definition of a virus. That is, a transmissible replication-competent intracellular parasite that causes the alleged novel disease 'COVID-19'. As was outlined in *The COVID-19 Fraud & War on Humanity*, there is no evidence that either the particle or the proposed novel disease exists.[179] Further, in this present essay there has been a more detailed breakdown of the Fan Wu et al. paper and their false claim regarding "identification" of a virus in Wuhan in early 2020. On the other hand, lab leak proponents such as Sachs and Harrison start their analysis by wholeheartedly accepting virology's unestablished premises.

In their paper they went on to cite aspects such as, "the collection of SARS-like bat CoVs from the field...[and]...the analysis and manipulation of these viruses," complaining that, "the precise nature of the experiments

---

[178] Neil Harrison and Jeffrey Sachs, "A call for an independent inquiry into the origin of the SARS-CoV-2 virus", *Proceedings of the National Academy of Sciences,* 19 May 2022: www.pnas.org/doi/abs/10.1073/pnas.2202769119

[179] Mark Bailey & John Bevan-Smith, "The COVID-19 Fraud & War on Humanity", 11 Nov 2021: https://drsambailey.com/covid-19/the-covid-19-fraud-war-on-humanity/

that were conducted, including the full array of viruses collected from the field and the subsequent sequencing and manipulation of those viruses, remains unknown." They obviously do not realise that 'SARS-like bat CoVs' are nothing more than ground up bat intestines, claimed to be "pathogenic" by injecting the muck directly into the brains of neonatal rats. Manipulation of such samples may be a way to secure some funding and impress the uninitiated but it does not change biological reality. Such experiments do not establish that their samples contain viruses or have any pathogenic properties in the natural world. If they can't even demonstrate the existence of viruses in their promoted public attempts, there is not much to worry about — it doesn't matter what goes on behind closed doors because they have no viruses to start with.

With regard to the 'SARS-CoV-2 genome' that the virologists have proffered, Sachs and Harrison stated they, "do not know whether the insertion of the FCS [furin[180] cleavage site] was the result of natural evolution - perhaps via a recombination event in an intermediate mammal or a human - or was the result of a deliberate introduction of the FCS into a SARS-like virus as part of a laboratory experiment." They would be better advised to look into how it was established that *any* of the sequences or proteins they are analysing belong to a pathogenic virus. The debate over the past few years concerning the intricacies of the FCS is simply a microcosm within the wider flawed paradigm of "viral" genomics and proteomics.

Similarly, their mention of alleged virus research taking place at the University of North Carolina (UNC) or "leaked" grant proposals such as "DEFUSE" made to the US Defense Advanced Research Projects Agency are not evidence of viruses.[181] To be clear, it is not being disputed that

---

[180] Furin is a protein-splitting enzyme that is present in humans and other animals. Virologists claim that when SARS-CoV-2 is being produced in a cell, furin cuts the spike protein at the 'furin cleavage site' before it exits the cell.

[181] Samantha Bailey, "Gain of Function Garbage", 18 Jan 2022: https://drsambailey.com/resources/videos/covid-19/gain-of-function-garbage/

institutions such as UNC have been experimenting with entities such as spike proteins for decades. Some of these sequences have been patented and used in the development of injectable biological agents, recently forced onto many people under the guise of COVID-19 vaccines.[182] However, none of this requires the existence of particles that qualify as viruses.

Unfortunately, virology's book of claims has become so convoluted that most readers do not realise that it is largely composed of nonsense. A few days after Sachs and Harrison published their article, *The Intercept* thought they were also on an investigative trail involving, "the intriguing theory of viral engineering."[183] They reported on a 2016 UNC Chapel Hill study[184] associated with Ralph Baric stating, "the scientists created a new virus using the spike of a bat coronavirus that had been isolated and characterized by the Wuhan Institute of Virology [WIV]." It can be safely assumed that the author does not appreciate how deceptively the virologists use the word 'isolated'. Additionally, Figure 1 on page 20 exposes the absurd claim that the WIV had "purified virions" that were then allegedly utilised by Baric et al. subsequently as they, "created a new virus." There was no evidence that either lab had anything more than abnormal monkey kidney cell culture soup.

The lab leak hypothesis is simply another narrative in the COVID-19 era that keeps alive in the public's imagination the illusion of the material existence of SARS-CoV-2, as well as pathogenic viruses and microbe-related contagion in general. In recent months the fear-based narrative has continued with declarations of monkeypox outbreaks, alleged

---

[182] Mark Bailey & John Bevan-Smith, "The COVID-19 Fraud & War on Humanity", 11 Nov 2021: https://drsambailey.com/covid-19/the-covid-19-fraud-war-on-humanity/

[183] Sharon Lerner, "Jeffrey Sachs presents evidence of possible lab origin of COVID-19", *The Intercept*, 20 May 2022: https://theintercept.com/2022/05/19/covid-lab-leak-evidence-jeffrey-sachs/

[184] Vineet Menachery, et al., "SARS-like WIV1-CoV poised for human emergence", *PNAS*, 14 Mar 2016: https://doi.org/10.1073/pnas.1517719113

detection of polio "viruses" in London, and the COVID-19 lab leak theory even received backing from the Director-General of the World Health Organization in support of the phantom disease and pandemic he named.[185] It seems likely there will be more "lab leak" stories in the future if they continue to capture attention so effectively.

Like the "Little Mountain Dog" story, the lab leak story doesn't rely on any scientific demonstration of a virus, it relies simply on the *belief* that there is a virus, aided by some apparent supporting evidence. Along the same lines, in November 2020, the Lowy Institute, which describes itself as an Australian "international policy think tank," published an article with the following introduction:

> *In April 2020 Dr Ai Fen, head of the emergency department at Wuhan Central Hospital, gave an interview to Chinese magazine Renwu. She described in great detail how, late in December 2019, she had begun receiving numerous patients into the emergency room with flu-like symptoms that were resistant to the usual treatments. She recounted how she "broke out in a cold sweat" when the first virus report of one of those patients came back. She hastily circled the words "SARS coronavirus", screen-shot the report, and sent it to colleagues. Very quickly, her report circulated around Wuhan medical circles. But instead of mobilising the hospital and authorities, Dr Ai's actions saw her reprimanded by the hospital disciplinary committee for "spreading rumours" and "harming stability". Rather than warning staff and the public, hospital authorities told staff not to wear personal protective equipment and relayed instructions from the local health protection committee that, to avoid causing panic, doctors*

[185] Mark Bailey, "Lab Leaks and other Legends", 28 Jun 2022: https://drsambailey.com/covid-19/lab-leaks-and-other-legends/

were prohibited from sharing messages and reports related to the virus.[186]

To the credulous it may sound like an attempt by the authorities to cover up the start of the "viral pandemic" but those familiar with virology's nonsense can see straight through the fallacies — none of this framing requires an actual virus. Circling 'SARS coronavirus' on a "virus report" is based on nothing more than what Fan Wu's and other teams have done in their dry-lab simulations.

Another doctor, Li Wenliang, hailed by the BBC as a "whistleblower,"[187] was also reported as being censored by the Chinese authorities after he shared Dr Ai's report. It was claimed that the 33-year-old Dr Li subsequently died of COVID-19 after he, "contracted the virus while working at Wuhan Central Hospital." The corporate media and Wikipedia's[188] lavish promotion of the "cover up" would be comedic if it wasn't part of a war against humanity. All of these stories lead back to the same fear narrative involving a contagious and "deadly virus." It allows this fraud to be propagated and paves the way for other similar frauds to be carried out in the future. It astounds the author that so many of the 'health freedom' community do not trust any of the corporate media's claims about COVID-19, *except* the declaration that a deadly virus is on the loose, the biggest lie of all.

The claim that "coronavirus" patent filings provide evidence that viruses exist can be dealt with briskly. In 2021, Dr David Martin of M·CAM® International, published, "The Fauci/COVID-19 Dossier,"[189] as part of the company's activities,

---

[186] Lydia Khalil, "Digital Authoritarianism, China and COVID", *Lowy Institute*, 2 Nov 2020: https://www.lowyinstitute.org/publications/digital-authoritarianism-china-and-covid

[187] "Li Wenliang: Coronavirus kills Chinese whistleblower doctor", *BBC*, 7 Feb 2020: https://www.bbc.com/news/world-asia-china-51403795

[188] "Li Wenliang", *Wikipedia*: https://en.wikipedia.org/wiki/Li_Wenliang

[189] David Martin, "The Fauci/COVID-19 Dossier" Apr 2021: https://www.davidmartin.world/wp-content/uploads/2021/01/The_Fauci_COVID-19_Dossier.pdf

monitoring possible violations of the 1925 Protocol for the Prohibition of the Use in War of Asphyxiating, Poisonous, or other Gases, and of Bacteriological Methods of Warfare (the Geneva Protocol) 1972 Convention on the Prohibition of the Development, Production, and Stockpiling of Bacteriological and Toxin Weapons and Their Destruction (the BTWC).

Despite the numerous patents involving, "methods for producing recombinant coronavirus," and federal grants to the likes of "gain of function specialist" Dr Ralph Baric and his team at UNC Chapel Hill, there is nothing in any of these documents that contain scientific evidence that viruses exist. Patent office staff and those approving research grants are not the arbiters of biological plausibility and simply carry forward the claims of the virologists. The dossier was no smoking gun for "gain of function" activities involving pathogenic viruses. Perhaps those thinking it was did not heed Martin's opening disclaimer that, "throughout this document, uses of terms commonly accepted in medical and scientific literature do not imply acceptance or rejection of the dogma that they represent."

VIROLOGY AND THE CLOSED SOCIETY

I'm not a scientist but it is the right and duty of every citizen to look and see what the scientists have said, and to analyse it for themselves, and to draw commonsense conclusions. We are all perfectly capable of doing that, and there's no particular reason why the scientific nature of the problem should mean that we have to resign our liberty into the hands of scientists.

— Lord Sumption, 2020.[190]

---

[190] Jonny Dymond interview of Lord Sumption, BBC Radio 4's *The World at One*, 30 Mar 2020. Transcript: https://www.conservativewoman.co.uk/a-hysterical-slide-into-a-police-state-judge-warns-of-liberty-being-forced-into-lockdown/

It was the United Kingdom's Health Security Agency (UKHSA) that provided one of the strangest responses ever seen with regard to concealing the true nature of supposed controls in their alleged "SARS-CoV-2 Isolation and Sequencing Experiments." On 27 October 2021, in relation to a Freedom of information request regarding virus isolation, they suggested that the image depicted in Figure 9 below provided "evidence" of the SARS-CoV-2 virus.[191] My colleague, who made the request, was not in the least bit fooled by a computer-generated image that came with no information as to the source of the image or how it was produced. The UKHSA continued to fumble with the science, stating that viruses, "require a host cell substrate to replicate. Isolation of any virus without any medium therefore is not possible...These media and any products added are all sterile and do not contain additional genetic material."[192] We can only speculate as to what the UKHSA think the host cells contain if not genetic material! Like the CDC, the response team also seemed to imply that the paper by Na Zhu et al., "A Novel Coronavirus from Patients with Pneumonia in China, 2019," provided reassurance that the imagined SARS-CoV-2 virus particle had a physical existence.

My colleague pointed out to the UKHSA that they had no proof of a virus and as such were implicating themselves by, "unnecessarily hurting everyone by instilling fear in them, summarily removing their rights, and coercing them into an unnecessary and harmful treatment which is morally reprehensible."[193] Undeterred, they wrote to the UKHSA again a few months later requesting disclosure of the complete methodology of the cell culture experiments and any comparative controls in the Public Health England paper, "Duration of infectiousness and correlation with RT-PCR cycle threshold values in cases of COVID-19, England, January to May

---

[191] (By email from Information Rights Team, UKHSA, "Case ref: 1409 - FOI Purification of SARS-CoV-2 and Variants (CF)", 27 Oct 2022.)

[192] Ibid.

[193] By email to UKHSA, "Case ref: 1409 - FOI Purification of SARS-CoV-2 and Variants (CF)", 27 Oct 2022.

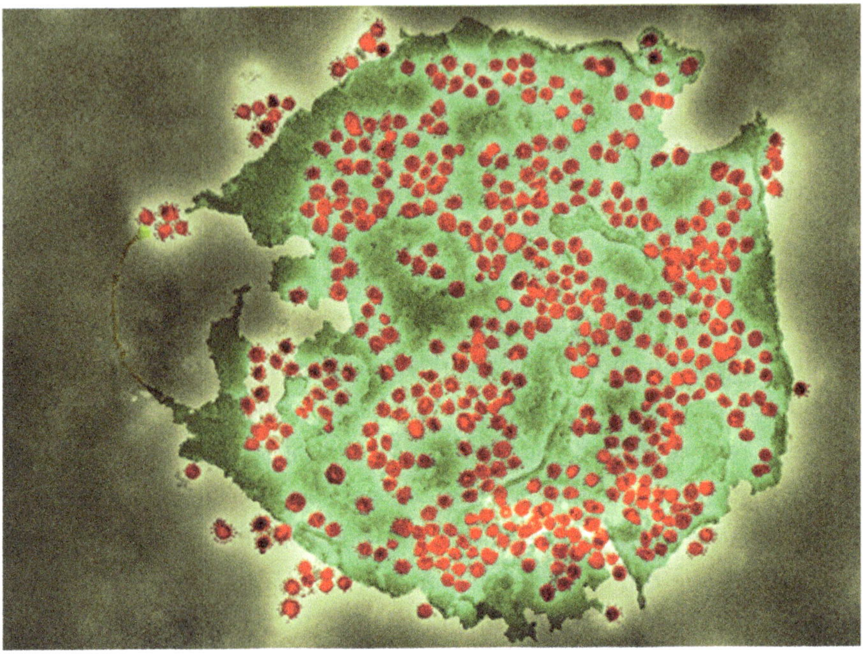

Figure 9. The UKHSA's farcical claimed "proof" of SARS-CoV-2 on 27 October 2021.

2020."[194] The response letter from the UKHSA dated 25 Mar 2022, contained text that represented either a conspiracy between the WHO and sovereign nation-states not to release details of the "viral culture" deception that lies at the heart of the COVID-19 fraud or a profound ignorance on the part of the UKHSA in describing SARS-CoV-2 as a "high hazard virus:"[195]

> *In accordance with Section 1(1)(a) of the Act, UKHSA can confirm that it holds the requested information pertaining to*

[194] Anika Singanayagam, et al., "Duration of infectiousness and correlation with RT-PCR cycle threshold values in cases of COVID-19, England, January to May 2020", *Euro Surveill,* 25(32), 13 Aug 2020: https://doi.org/10.2807/1560-7917.ES.2020.25.32.2001483

[195] The UKHSA themselves had declared that "as of 19 March 2020, COVID-19 is no longer considered to be a high consequence infectious disease (HCID) in the UK.": https://www.gov.uk/guidance/high-consequence-infectious-diseases-hcid

the above questions. However, the information requested is exempt from disclosure in accordance with the Section 24(1) - National Security exemption. Section 24(1) provides that information is exempt if exemption from Section 1(1)(b) is required for the purposes of safeguarding national security. Whereby, required is taken to mean that the use of the exemption is reasonably necessary...

Factors supporting maintaining the exemption include:

- *Disclosure of information would constitute very detailed technical information, transferring know how, which would directly contravene an explicit request from the World Health Organization (WHO) to Public Health England (PHE now UKHSA) in 2020 not to release or make widely available the details of culture amplification of SARS-CoV-2;*
- *Disclosure of this would be the detailing of exact methodology utilised in virus amplification for a designated high hazard virus, requiring containment Level 3 and could pose a threat to national and global biosecurity if provided to an unascertained or unvetted member of the public or agents with ill intent;*
- *Disclosure of this information would provide a significant "know how" capability that could in some circumstances be considered a biosecurity threat.*[196]

A review of this decision was requested by my colleague but the decision was upheld by the UKHSA on 3 May 2022, on the grounds that providing the details of the cell culture experiment, "was outweighed by the national security threat that the disclosure poses."[197] It is unclear why keeping the details of their experimental methodology under wraps is

---

[196] Letter from UKHSA, "25/01/2022/ag/2334, Re: FOIA: SARS-CoV-2 Isolation and Sequencing Experiments' Controls", 25 Mar 2022: https://www.fluoridefreepeel.ca/wp-content/uploads/2022/05/UK-HSA-isolation-sequencing-methods-PACKAGE-redacted.pdf

[197] Letter from UKHSA, "01/0422/ag/005, Re: Case ref 2334 - FOIA: SARS-CoV-2 Isolation and Sequencing Experiments' Controls", 3 May 2022.

necessary for the UK's efforts in "safeguarding national security." It has been exposed that the virologists are not performing valid control experiments and their claims of "isolating viruses" have not been established in the scientific literature. Are the authorities worried that if they officially admit as much, there will be a revolt when the wider public realise the crimes that have been carried out on the basis of claims stemming from fraudulent virological experiments? Their official obstruction of the release of this information to the public, citing "biosecurity", is paradoxical given that the alleged "high hazard virus" cannot be shown to exist.

The asinine responses from the UKHSA were perhaps only topped by Maggie Throup, the Parliamentary Under Secretary of State for Vaccines and Public Health. In an email to fellow MP Rachael Maskell on 27 June 2022, Throup stated that,

> *"the UK Health Security Agency (UKHSA) does not use Koch's postulates in COVID-19, as they are too limiting, suggesting association more than causation. Koch also dropped his postulates when he discovered asymptomatic carriage. The Bradford-Hill criteria are more commonly used when associating a virus and disease. However, it should be noted that, SARS-CoV-2 fulfils Koch's postulates as demonstrated in the following paper where [an] animal model has been used."*[198]

As was outlined earlier in this section of the essay, it is absurd to claim the postulates could be fulfilled when the existence of the postulated microbe was never established. Additionally, the 2020 paper Throup refers to is, "The pathogenicity of SARS-CoV-2 in hACE2 transgenic mice."[199] This paper

---

198 By email from Maggie Throup MP to Rachael Maskell MP, Ref: ZA50772, 27 June 2022: https://www.parallelparliament.co.uk/question/315/coronavirus

199 Linlin Bao, et al., "The pathogenicity of SARS-CoV-2 in hACE2 transgenic mice", *Nature*, 7 May 2020: https://www.nature.com/articles/s41586-020-2312-y

never established that there was a virus in their samples, had no valid controls, did not follow Koch's postulates, and exhibited other aspects of fraud.[200] However, Throup then continued to promote virological nonsense claiming that another study,[201] "demonstrates the course of COVID-19 disease, from the moment a person first encountered SARS-CoV-2, throughout the infection to the point at which the virus is apparently eliminated." Once again, the paper simply asserted there was a virus in their samples and had no valid controls, not to mention the other unscientific aspects of the study that have been dealt with elsewhere, including *ViroLIEgy*'s comprehensive refutation of the paper while it was a preprint.[202] In other words, politicians such as Throup are parroting virology's nonsense and thereby subjecting their constituents to an obscene range of unnecessary and sometimes deadly consequences.

METAGENOMIC SEQUENCING — VIROLOGY'S FINAL GASP?

> *Is the reductionist ambition for molecular biology in danger of being thwarted by the volume of the data it produces, or even by the absorbing interest of its collection?*
>
> — Sir John Maddox[203]

The cost of sequencing has fallen dramatically since 2001, when it was over US$5000 per raw megabase (Mb), through to 2007 when it was around $500 per Mb, after which it dropped precipitously to $0.005 per

---

[200] Samantha Bailey, "Koch's Postulates: Germ School Dropout", 8 Sep 2022: https://drsambailey.com/resources/videos/germ-theory/kochs-postulates-germ-school-dropout/

[201] Ben Killingley, et al., "Safety, tolerability and viral kinetics during SARS-CoV-2 human challenge in young adults", *Nat Med*, 31 Mar 2022: https://pubmed.ncbi.nlm.nih.gov/35361992/

[202] Mike Stone, "Challenging 'SARS-COV-2'", 11 Feb 2022: https://viroliegy.com/2022/02/11/challenging-sars-cov-2/

[203] "Finding wood among the trees", *Nature*, 5 May 1988: https://www.nature.com/articles/333011a0.pdf

Mb by mid-2021.[204] Additionally, the emergence of Next Generation Sequencing (NGS) around 2005 resulted in a massive reduction in the time required to sequence genomes. As stated in a 2017 *Biology and Medicine* paper,

> *the human genome, for example, consists of 3 billion bps* [base pairs]...*the sequencing of the human genome using the Sanger sequencing took almost 15 years, required the cooperation of many laboratories around the world and costed approximately 100 million US dollars, whereas the sequencing by NGS sequencers using the 454 Genome Sequencer FLX took two months and for approximately one hundredth of the cost.*[205]

The same paper went on to state, "unfortunately, NGS are incapable [*sic*] to read the complete DNA sequence of the genome, they are limited to sequence small DNA fragments and generate millions of reads. This limit remains a negative point especially for genome assembly projects because it requires high computing resources."

It is pointed out that with regard to virology, a far bigger concern than "computing resources" is that a process that can be employed for sequencing genetic material of known provenance (e.g. human, bacterial, and fungal cells) has morphed into algorithmic assembly of genetic fragments of unknown provenance. This is the virus hunters' basis of identifying what they claim are viruses. Computing resources are no longer a problem for the virologists as they mine information from their completely anti-scientific "wet-lab pipeline" methodologies involving

---

[204] National Human Genome Research Institute, "DNA Sequencing Costs: Data": https://www.genome.gov/about-genomics/fact-sheets/DNA-Sequencing-Costs-Data (accessed 23 Apr 2022).

[205] Mehdi Kchouk, et al., "Generations of Sequencing Technologies: From First to Next Generation", *Biology and Medicine*, 6 Mar 2017: https://www.walshmedicalmedia.com/abstract/generations-of-sequencing-technologies-from-first-to-next-generation-24326.html

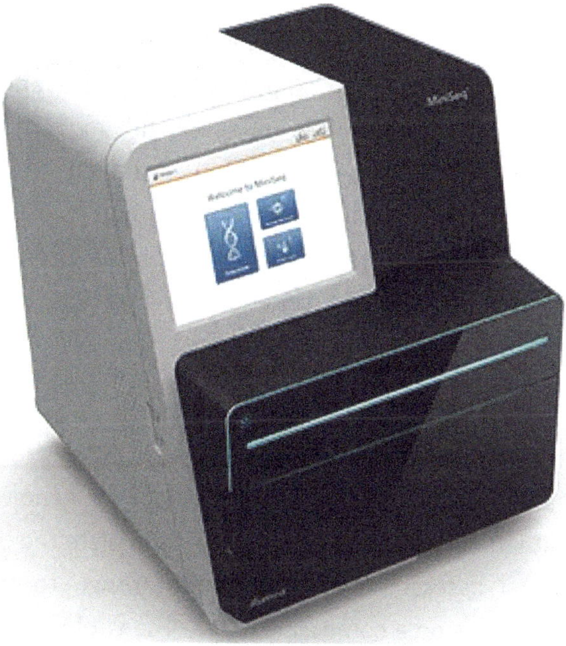

Figure 10. The *Illumina MiniSeq* system - how Fan Wu's team and others find *in silico* "viruses" in the 21st century through computational algorithms. It takes place in the dry-lab pipeline without demonstrating the existence of an actual infectious disease-causing particle.

crude samples and feed these generated unfiltered reads into their theoretical "dry-lab pipeline" and its *in silico* models.

It would seem that the combination of massively reduced sequencing costs and shortened time frames have accelerated the descent of virology into further anti-science, for which humanity is paying a very dear price for non-existent viruses that are invented at will and used as excuses for spurious interventions and enslavement. An October 2019 publication in *Critical Reviews in Microbiology* claimed that, "mNGS [metagenomic NGS] performs well in identifying rare, novel, difficult-to-detect and co-infected pathogens directly from clinical samples."[206] However, "performs well" with regards to identifying novel "viral pathogens" is meaningless as they too have fallen into virology's circular reasoning vortex. Most of the "novel pathogens" they listed in their paper were viruses derived from the purportedly advantageous "culture-independent" modern technique of mNGS. Once again however, if nobody can culture or physically isolate alleged viruses, how can various genetic sequences in environmental samples be claimed to come from them? As has been outlined, the declaration by Fan Wu et al. of a "new coronavirus" in Wuhan was based entirely on such proffered genetic sequences. Virology's attempt to pass off this methodology as proof of virus particles has introduced an unfalsifiable hypothesis that is inconsistent with the scientific method.

The specialisation (and increasing automation) of the genomics process is leading to a situation where few people can appreciate the overall picture from the clinical assessment of a patient through to the generated nucleotide sequences on a computer screen. The virologists invalidate the 'virus genome' process from step one by never establishing that they have a particle that meets the definition of a virus. They certainly never demonstrate that the sequences they claim are 'viral' come from inside such an imagined particle. Instead they claim that such declarations can be made by consensus decisions, whether the sequences are labelled 'non-human' or 'novel' and by how much they happen to match 'known viral' sequences that were previously deposited on the genetic databanks. However, nature does not obey stories created by mankind.

The metagenomics process allows for the *de novo* invention of such viral sequences and has allowed virology's merry-go-round to keep spinning into the 21st century. However, due to the inability of virology to fulfil its own postulates for the past century, its future is almost certainly going to be built entirely around this misuse, or at least misapplication, of

---

[206] Donsheng Han, et al., "mNGS in clinical microbiology laboratories: on the road to maturity", *Critical Reviews in Microbiology*, 6 Nov 2019: https://doi.org/10.1080/1040841X.2019.1681933

metagenomics. One might hope that the recent failure of multiple organisations to prove they are performing valid control experiments indicates that viral pandemics are on their last legs scientifically. They can only be propagated for as long as this final fraud is hidden from the public. It could be expected in virology's final gasp, metagenomics will continue to be deceptively sold as a 'technological advancement' conveniently claimed to have rendered the proper scientific proofs obsolete.

As has been outlined, the follies of such 'technological advancement' can usually be exposed with one simple question to check if is adhering to the scientific method. For example, in 2020, a Canadian team claimed that they were comparing various techniques for, "whole genome sequencing of SARS-CoV-2," from nasal swabs taken from two individuals alleged to have COVID-19.[207] One of the authors was Dr Andrew McArthur, an associate professor of biochemistry and biomedical sciences at McMaster University, Canada. He was asked if they, "[tried] to extract RNA from healthy controls (healthy persons or PCR-negative samples) or from uninfected supernatant but virus-free," to see if they could also assemble a "SARS-CoV-2 genome" through their methodology? McArthur responded that, "we did not have swabs from healthy controls but the study included negative controls for application/libraries, i.e. no sample RNA included."[208] Indeed, there was only one mention of a 'control' in the paper where it stated, "a negative control library with no input SARS-CoV-2 RNA extract was included using ARTIC amplification." Once again, the lack of a valid control, being a human-derived sample *sans* the alleged "virus," places this paper in the extensive archives of virology's metagenomic nonsense. Ironically, their paper also claimed that, "COVID-19 is caused by severe acute respiratory syndrome coronavirus 2

---

[207] Jalees Nasir, et al., "A Comparison of Whole Genome Sequencing of SARS-CoV-2 Using Amplicon-Based Sequencing, Random Hexamers, and Bait Capture", *Viruses*, 15 Aug 2020: https://www.mdpi.com/1999-4915/12/8/895

[208] By email from Andrew McArthur, 31 May 2022: https://www.fluoridefreepeel.ca/wp-content/uploads/2022/06/Mubareka-Mossman-etc-no-valid-controls-PACKAGE-redacted.pdf

(SARS-CoV-2), a novel coronavirus, which emerged in December 2019," with the citation being the Peng Zhou et al. paper, the fraud of which was exposed earlier in this essay.

WHY QUESTION VIRUS EXISTENCE DURING A WAR?

The author has observed and been in contact with a number of individuals in the 'health freedom' movement who contest that it is pointless to entertain discussions concerning whether SARS-CoV-2 or any other pathogenic viruses have been shown to exist. Some of the arguments that have been advanced include that it distracts from the crimes being committed against humanity, that it is a strategic mistake as it causes more division, and that if the viral hypothesis (or wider germ "theory") is being disputed then an alternative theory must be presented. There is no need to provide a laundry list of individuals advancing such claims but one example was British academic Dr Roger Watson who stated in March 2022, "it is hard to understand how Sam Bailey arrives at her views and it is not necessary to be a virus denier to be highly critical of the way the pandemic was managed."[209] Watson's criticism exemplifies what is hoped to have been shown as an ill-informed opinion that relies on parroting virology's claims. Our views should not be hard to understand for those who have extensively investigated the history, anti-scientific methodologies and pronouncements of the virologists, including the declaration of a "novel coronavirus" in 2020, and made efforts to communicate this fraud to the public in plain language.

In some cases these critics state that everything about the pandemic is a fraud, *except* the claim by the virologists (and the WHO) that SARS-CoV-2 has a physical existence as a pathogenic particle. They cannot see that the very basis of the fraud is also a fraud. The difficulty for some, even those in the freedom movement, could be that the repudiation of virus

[209] Samantha Bailey, "The COVID 'Sceptics' Who Spread Viral Dogma", 17 Mar 2022: https://drsambailey.com/covid-19/the-covid-sceptics-who-spread-viral-dogma/

existence would come at the cost of calling into question much of their life's work. However, during an investigation one should not stop for reasons of convenience or because one's current state of knowledge goes no further. On the contrary, it is a grave mistake to allow the foundational "facts" to be dictated by the virology establishment. The heart of the COVID-19 fraud is based on virology's claims. It is not a strategic mistake to direct our energy towards exposing virology's fallacies, otherwise defeating COVID-19 responses while leaving the virological nonsense intact opens the door to any number of "viral pandemics" in the future. Gaining insight into the entire fraud eliminates the unfounded fear of contagion and equips one with a more robust path to enduring freedom.

POSTSCRIPT

No matter how long an essay covering this topic may be, there will always be more questions in the form of, "but what about...?" The desire to fit observed phenomena to the virus model is strongly programmed on many levels. It was not the intention of this essay to explain peripheral observations or the cause of various illnesses in organisms such as humans. As has been detailed, it only needs to be demonstrated that the viral hypothesis has refuted itself on its own terms. The virologists have provided no direct evidence of pathogenic viruses and instead have resorted to indirect observations that are invalid due to the uncontrolled nature of the experiments. Additionally, adhering to the scientific method places us under no obligation to provide an alternative explanation for these phenomena — when a hypothesis has been falsified, even once, it is done for. Tragically, the explanations to many of the "but what about...?" questions have already been answered elsewhere but the seduction of the "virus" and the juggernaut of surrounding interests have formed an artificial knowledge barrier for many people. In this light, I have endeavoured to serve the highest purpose I know and hope that my contributions will help humanity throw off the imaginary viral shackles once and for all.

Progress consists, not in the increase of truth, but in freeing it from its wrappings. The truth is obtained like gold, not by letting it grow bigger, but by washing off from it everything that isn't gold.

— Leo Tolstoy[210]

[210] *Tolstoy's Diaries*, edited and translated by R. F. Christian, Flamingo, 1994.

ADDITIONAL ESSAYS

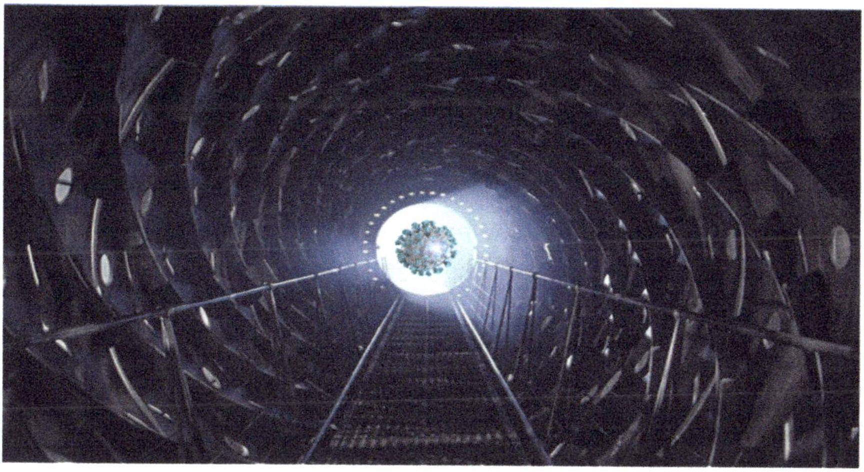

1. VIROLOGY'S EVENT HORIZON

31st of March, 2024

A commentary on why the virologists cannot perform valid control experiments with their cell culture techniques. The purported 'gold standard' evidence for "viruses" has a fundamental logical flaw and the methodology cannot establish whether hypothesised particles exist in nature.

The pursuit of virology has come under intense scrutiny since early 2020. This was precipitated by the onset of the COVID-19 era, particularly when the World Health Organization's Director-General, Dr. Tedros Adhanom Ghebreyesus, stood in front of the international media on the 11th of March, 2020, and stated, "COVID-19 can be characterized as a pandemic."[211] For many people, the fraud of the alleged pandemic started around that time or during the subsequent lockdowns and severe restrictions on freedom of movement and civil rights. For others the fraud started in 2009 when the WHO changed the definition of 'pandemic' and

---

[211] Ghebreyesus, T., "WHO Director-General's opening remarks at the media briefing on COVID-19 - 11 March 2020," 11 Mar 2020: https://www.who.int/director-general/speeches/detail/who-director-general-s-opening-remarks-at-the-media-briefing-on-covid-19---11-march-2020 (archived)

the words, "with enormous numbers of deaths and illness" were suddenly excluded from the existing meaning.[212]

We have pointed out that although the above-mentioned developments appear fraudulent, they were simply smaller offshoots of a foundational scientific fraud known as 'virological science'.[213, 214, 215] These lesser offshoots can be referred to as "downstream" aspects that become logically redundant when the premises upon which they relied are presently shown to be non-existent or at the least, apparently unverifiable hypotheses.

So what is the alleged scientific evidence that underpins the concept of a 'pandemic' regardless of the shade in which it is being painted? And how does its subsequent examination disqualify virology as a science?

Online encyclopaedia *Wikipedia* states that a pandemic is, "an **epidemic** of an **infectious disease** that has spread across a large region, for instance multiple continents or worldwide, affecting a substantial number of individuals."[216] (emphasis added) An epidemic is defined as, "the rapid spread of disease to a large number of hosts in a given population within a short period of time."[217] An infectious disease is one that involves, "the invasion of tissues by **pathogens**, their multiplication, and the reaction of host tissues to the **infectious agent** and the toxins they produce."[218]

---

212 Law, R., "WHO and the pandemic flu 'conspiracies'", 6 Jun 2020: https://www.bmj.com/rapid-response/2011/11/02/who-changed-definition-influenza-pandemic

213 Engelbrecht, T., et al., *Virus Mania*, 3rd English Edition, Books on Demand, 2021: https://drsambailey.com/shop-2/

214 Bailey, M. & Bevan-Smith, J., *The COVID-19 Fraud & War on Humanity*, 11 Nov 2021: https://drsambailey.com/the-covid-19-fraud-war-on-humanity/

215 Bailey, M., *A Farewell to Virology (Expert Edition)*, 15 Sep 2022: https://drsambailey.com/a-farewell-to-virology-expert-edition/

216 "Pandemic," *Wikipedia*: https://en.wikipedia.org/wiki/Pandemic (accessed 10 Mar 2024)

217 "Epidemic," *Wikipedia*: https://en.wikipedia.org/wiki/Epidemic (accessed 10 Mar 2024)

218 "Infection," *Wikipedia*: https://en.wikipedia.org/wiki/Infection (accessed 10 Mar 2024)

(emphasis added) Furthermore, it is stated that, "an infectious disease, also known as a transmissible disease or communicable disease, is an illness resulting from an infection."[219]

These alleged "pathogens" include viruses which are said to be submicroscopic particles that have specific physical and biological properties, including replication-competence and the ability to transmit between organisms such as humans to cause disease. (The arguments about whether they are true micro-organisms, dead or alive, etc are further downstream considerations and of no consequence compared to the pivotal question of their existence.) While many people take the existence of viruses as an established scientific fact, my experience indicates that most people, including those in the health community, have not critically examined the cited evidence to verify for themselves whether the relevant methodologies that were utilised qualify as scientific. It also remains largely unappreciated that viruses were not discovered and then studied - they were *imagined*. Virology went on to invent itself on the basis of these *hypothetical* particles:

> *...one of the pivotal issues with virology was that it invented itself as a field before establishing if viruses actually existed. It has been trying to justify itself since its inception: In this instance, a virus particle was not observed first and subsequently viral theory and pathology developed. Scientists of the mid and late nineteenth century were preoccupied with the identification of imagined contagious pathogenic entities...The extant presupposition of the time was that a very small germ particle existed that may explain contagion. What came thereafter arose to fulfil the presuppositional premise.*[220]

---

[219] Ibid.

[220] Bailey, M., *A Farewell to Virology (Expert Edition)*, 15 Sep 2022: https://drsambailey.com/a-farewell-to-virology-expert-edition/

What has taken place for over a century has been a series of pseudoscientific practices, including the continued use of a reification fallacy - that is, assuming viruses have a physical existence despite the fact that they remain a hypothetical construct. In other words, "the error of treating something that is not concrete, such as an idea, as a concrete thing."[221]

It can be shown that the virologists have painted themselves into a corner and the paradigm that they have created has them snared. If the discipline of virology is said to be a branch of natural science, then its practitioners are reliant on empirical evidence gained through observation and experimentation. Within this framework of the scientific method lies the requirement to generate a hypothesis (that is necessarily falsifiable) and then to test it with experiments. The experiments in question must possess a dependent variable, the part that is an observation or effect that depends on an independent variable. The independent variable is the postulated cause of this observation or effect. Experiments also require a 'control', namely the ability to compare variables and conditions in a manner that makes it possible to observe the results when varying *one* factor at a time.

There can be no excuse for allowing virologists to depart from the scientific field they claim to be operating within. As was noted in *A Farewell to Virology (Expert Edition)*:

> *In 2008, the journal Infection and Immunity featured a guest commentary titled, "Descriptive Science" that explained why, "descriptive research by itself is seldom conclusive," and may simply serve as a starting point to orientate further investigations. The authors pointed out that, "microbiology and immunology are now experimental sciences and*

---

[221] "Reification (fallacy)", *Wikipedia*: https://en.wikipedia.org/wiki/Reification_(fallacy) (accessed 10 Mar 2024)

> *consequently investigators can go beyond simply describing observations to formulate hypotheses and then perform experiments to validate or refute them."*[222]

And herein lies the complete downfall of virology and the virus model itself. An experiment that follows the scientific method and purports to show the *existence* of a virus needs to have a valid control to establish that the observed effects are the result of the virus (the claimed independent variable) and not other factors.

If the virologists even attempt to perform a control experiment in their methodologies they assert to demonstrate viral existence, frequently omitted are the details of the "mock-infected" group in their publications. The definition of mock-infected is:

> *...a control group in scientific experiments designed to evaluate the effects of viral infection on cells or organisms. In a mock-infected control group, the cells or organisms are* ***treated with the same conditions and reagents as the infected group, except they are not exposed to the virus.***[223] (emphasis added)

> *A control used in infection experiments. Two specimens are used one that is infected with the virus/vector of interest the other is* ***treated the same way except without the virus.***[224] (emphasis added)

[222] Bailey, M., *A Farewell to Virology (Expert Edition)*, 15 Sep 2022: https://drsambailey.com/a-farewell-to-virology-expert-edition/

[223] "mock-infected," *GenScript*: https://www.genscript.com/biology-glossary/10558/mock-infected

[224] "mock-infected," NW University: https://groups.molbiosci.northwestern.edu/holmgren/Glossary/Definitions/Def-M/mock-infected.html

In other words, the only difference for the control group is *one* variable - the alleged virus. This can be done in the case of bacterial or fungal cells because it is possible to separate out such cells and leave the other biological material in the sample.[*225]

It is therefore contested that the virologists themselves have conceded that a true mock-infected experiment is an impossibility as apparently they cannot physically isolate (and thus remove) virus particles from specimens derived from an organism said to be afflicted by a "viral" illness.[*226] Thus, the only experiments they can possibly perform must fall back on the prior *assertion* that viral particles are present in one group and not present in the 'mock-infected' group. It is a logical fallacy in the form of *petitio principii*, also known as 'begging the question' in that it purports to prove a proposition while simultaneously taking the proposition for granted.[227, *228]

Although many of us that have criticised the virus model have noted this problem before,[229] we have perhaps not been explicit enough in pointing out that the reason the virologists have "neglected" to perform valid cell

---

225 *There is no evidence that any micro-organisms *per se* have "pathogenic" abilities to invade healthy tissue and cause disease: https://drsambailey.com/resources/videos/germ-theory/why-pathogens-dont-exist/, however experiments with valid controls are possible with bacterial and fungal cells so the hypothesis can be tested.

226 *As of the 23rd of March, 2024, biostatistician Christine Massey has collated official responses from 222 medical and science institutions confirming that none have evidence of the alleged 'SARS-CoV-2' virus ever being found in a human: https://www.fluoridefreepeel.ca/fois-reveal-that-health-science-institutions-around-the-world-have-no-record-of-sars-cov-2-isolation-purification/ (accessed 30 Mar 2024)

227 Welton, J., *A manual of logic, Volume 2*, 1905: "*Petitio principii* is, therefore, committed when a proposition which requires proof is assumed without proof.": https://archive.org/details/amanuallogicvol00weltgoog/page/n298/mode/2up

228 *There are in fact two instances of the *petitio principii* fallacy being committed during the cell culture process: the first is that viruses are present in the 'viral illness' sample and the second is that no viruses are present in the 'mock-infected' sample. This essay outlines why *neither* determination can be made by the cell culture technique.

229 Cowan, T., et al., "The 'Settling The Virus Debate' Statement," 14 Jul 2022: https://drsambailey.com/resources/settling-the-virus-debate/

culture control experiments is because that, by definition, they are not able to do so.*[230]

Their predicament goes deeper than the attempts to physically isolate particles derived from the procedure of "culturing" hypothesised viruses during *in vitro* experiments.*[231] Once again, this practice is scientifically invalid as a methodology to establish the *existence* of something because the interpretation of the results depends entirely upon the presumption that the 'something' must exist. Cytopathic effects (CPEs) are claimed to indicate the presence of viruses but they can only be said to be the

230 *Critics of the cell culture technique have stated that control experiments have occasionally been performed and as they also produced cytopathic effects this refuted the virologists' own experiment. (For example in this video that analysed John Enders' 1954 'Cytopathogenic Agents from Measles Cases' paper, @1.18.25 https://odysee.com/@spacebusters:c9/Final-The-End-of-Germ-Theory:8) However, the analysis neglects the correct definition of 'mock-infected'. In order to be properly controlled in this setting there needs to be manipulation of *one* independent variable (the "cytopathogenic agent" or "virus"), something that the virologists are unable to do as this essay outlines. The presence or absence of the disease of measles said to be exhibited by a patient is not an independent variable in the laboratory experiment. Additionally, Enders stated in the 1954 paper that, "**a second agent** was obtained from an uninoculated culture of monkey kidney cells," implying that a different "virus" was already present in the cell line or had contaminated that particular culture. This "virus" was reported to produce distinct cytopathic effects: "when the cells from infected cultures were fixed and stained, their effect could be **easily distinguished** since the inter-nuclear changes typical of the measles agents were not observed." Thus it was never considered to be a control and the technique could be "maintained" on these terms. Despite Enders clearly not having a valid control (nor could he) the author would agree that it is still further evidence against the utility of the cell culture technique. See also note 228 for the fatal logical flaw in the cell culture technique *regardless* of the results.

231 *The virologists have failed on this front as well: they have not produced evidence that any "purified" particles derived from cell cultures can satisfy Koch's or Rivers' postulates for pathogenicity. Furthermore, the introduction of "sequence-based identification of microbial pathogens" by Fredricks and Relman in 1997 cannot be used to establish the existence of viruses and the authors themselves conceded that, "with only amplified sequence available, the biological role or even existence of these inferred microorganisms remains unclear.": https://europepmc.org/backend/ptpmcrender.fcgi?accid=PMC172879&blobtype=pdf In any case, note 225 outlines the foundational issue: the scientifically-formulated Koch's postulates were never demonstrated for any microbe, even those that can be shown to exist. See also https://drsambailey.com/resources/videos/germ-theory/kochs-postulates-germ-school-dropout/ and https://drsambailey.com/resources/videos/germ-theory/tb-cows-lies-and-koch-ups/

observation of cells breaking down in a test well. The CPEs are the dependent variable in the experiment but it is patently clear that no independent variable (a "virus") can be discerned in this process. The postulated virus remains hypothetical as it could not be identified as a specific entity at the start of the procedure and cannot then be claimed to have a physical existence based solely on subsequent observations involving the dependent variable.

At this point, it may be claimed that the *in vitro* appearance of vesicular nanoparticles in a cell culture mixed with a specimen derived from an organism with a "viral" illness provides evidence that viruses exist. However, this once again invokes the aforementioned *petitio principii* fallacy as the existence of a virus (and many of its hypothesised properties) is asserted in advance in the form of the "viral" illness.

We can summarise that some of the problems with using cell cultures as purported evidence include:

(a) The particles being declared as "viral" are seen for the first time as part of the CPE observations, i.e. they are dependent variables. It is preposterous to claim that they are also *the* independent variable in the same experiment.

(b) The *in vitro* (laboratory) observations cannot be known to replicate an *in vivo* (within living) process.[232]

(c) The techniques involved in electron microscopy introduce further variables that are not controlled, in addition to technical artefact and the further limitation that they are static structures embedded in resin, not living tissue.[233, 234]

---

232 Bailey, S., "Electron Microscopy and Unidentified 'Viral' Objects," 16 Feb 2022: https://drsambailey.com/resources/videos/covid-19/electron-microscopy-and-unidentified-viral-objects/

233 Ibid.

234 Hillman, H., *Certainty & Uncertainty in Biochemical Techniques*, Surrey University Press, U.K, 1972. For a summary see here: https://www.big-lies.org/harold-hillman-biology/certainty-and-uncertainty-in-biochemical-techniques.htm

The details of each published cell culture experiment can be analysed in depth; something that has been done by us and others on numerous occasions.*[235] In themselves, points (b) and (c) raise currently insurmountable problems as it is unclear if the observations in these settings replicate natural biology. Regardless, the entire process relies on a logical fallacy, a manifestation of which is expressed in point (a) and with regard to the pivotal virus existence question it renders the entire exercise invalid.

Keep in mind that the cell culture technique is virology's 'gold standard' of evidence that has been advanced to *establish* the postulated virus model. Whether any of the practitioners have realised that the methodology they have employed could not possibly be scientifically controlled is unknown. The crucial premise of the virus definition is pathogenic particles that *cause* replica particles in a host but the established 'gold standard' cell cultures cannot make a determination of their *existence* - the information is beyond the technique's "event horizon". By all accounts, there is nothing left to fall back upon and no escape from such a redundant paradigm.

The virologists may protest that these techniques are the only ones at their disposal because it is not possible to obtain the hypothesised viruses directly from living humans or other organisms, something that they once set out to do but apparently abandoned. Such a protest is of no scientific merit and the burden of proof remains squarely on their shoulders. The attempts to support the virus model through scientific methods have clearly failed and the imagined viruses have no known existence outside of logical fallacies and pseudoscientific claims.

---

[235] *Among the other questionable elements in the cell culture techniques employed by the virologists is the selection of cell lines that may be: (a) unrelated to the diseased cell type in the organism, (b) chromosomally abnormal, and (c) from another species. In further circular reasoning, it is conspicuous that such cells have been chosen because they have a propensity to react in the way desired by the virologists. Fatally for the technique, it has also been shown that CPEs can be a result of the process itself with no introduction of external specimens: https://drsambailey.com/a-farewell-to-virology-expert-edition/

The citation of indirect observations such as clinical conditions, apparent clusters of illness, antibody assays, genomics, proteomics and tests such as the polymerase chain reaction cannot stand as evidence of viruses because the claimant is starting within a loop of circular reasoning in which they have already assumed virus existence. None of these observations can possibly provide the required evidence to verify the virus model. The original sin involved the reification fallacy. Unfortunately for humanity, the virologists' imaginings about their particles spread to enough minds to bring the world to its knees in 2020.*[236] A petard has been created but who will it ultimately hoist?

For 'tis the sport to have the enginer
Hoist with his own petard; and 't shall go hard[237]

[236] *The presumption of "viral" illnesses and contagiousness is part of a trail of suffering induced by the conviction that 'germs' cause disease. This history of misplaced beliefs is outlined in *The Final Pandemic - An Antidote to Medical Tyranny*, 2024, particularly chapters 2 and 3: https://drsambailey.com/the-final-pandemic/

[237] Shakespeare, W., *The Tragedy of Hamlet, Prince of Denmark*, 1603

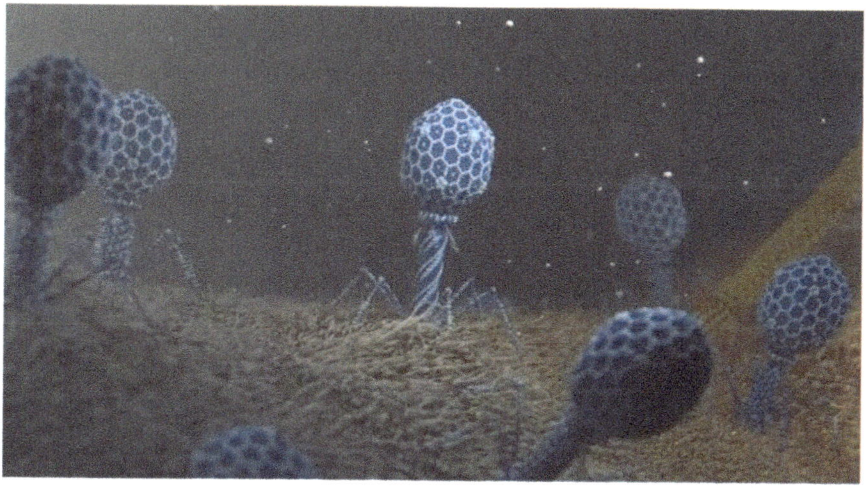

2. VIRUS, BACTERIOPHAGE & SINGLE "VIRUS" GENOMICS

20th of July, 2024

While the notional virus model has changed over time, the underlying premise of a contagious disease-causing entity has never been established. Nevertheless, its proponents have attempted to incorporate naturally-observed particles such as "bacteriophages" into the virological realm without establishing they are viruses, while portraying technological advances as the reason for their purported discovery. Single "virus" genomics is yet another chapter in the technology-driven world of virology that remains embedded within a flawed model.

Virus

The concept and meaning of 'virus' have been through a number of iterations over several hundred years. The appearance of the word in the English language in the 14th century derived from the Latin *virus* meaning, "poison, sap of plants, slimy liquid, a potent juice".[238] It is said that the reference to an "agent that causes infectious disease" had emerged by the 1790s and the modern scientific use commenced in the 1880s.[239] From

---

238 https://www.etymonline.com/search?q=virus

239 Ibid.

the first purported discovery of a virus there has been no consistent definition of what a virus is because, unlike other empirical biological sciences, there has never been a tangible viral particle that could be naturally observed, described, isolated, characterized and tested for pathogenicity. Hence, without a tangible asset for virologists to engage with, the term virus has taken on a protean quality, shimmying its way from one prêt-à-porter definition to the next in order to keep up with the latest viral theory.*[240]

A pervasive theme in virology's development is that the notion of some invisible contagious entity was *imagined* and then subsequent indirect observations have been advanced to support the hypothesized entity. On this timeline, the tobacco mosaic virus was allegedly the first virus discovered in the 1890s. However, neither that first purported discovery nor any purported discovery since has demonstrated any "virus" that is consistent with the modern definition: a particle that is disease-causing, replication-competent and contagious through natural exposure routes.[241, 242] (The imagined transmissible particle itself is known as a 'virion'.*[243])

The Dutch microbiologist Martinus Beijerinck used the term *contagium vivum fluidum* or "contagious living fluid" in the title of his 1898 paper concerning the cause of tobacco mosaic disease.[244] He proposed it related

---

240 *Dr John Bevan-Smith in private correspondence with the author, 9 Jul 2024.

241 Bailey, S., "Tobacco Mosaic 'Virus' – The beginning & end of virology," *drsambailey.com*, 5 Apr 2022: https://drsambailey.com/resources/videos/viruses-unplugged/tobacco-mosaic-virus-the-beginning-and-end-of-virology/

242 Bailey, M., *A Farewell to Virology (Expert Edition)*, 15 Sep 2022: https://drsambailey.com/a-farewell-to-virology-expert-edition/

243 *"Jean-Michel Claverie pointed out that the viral factory corresponds to the real viral organism, whereas the virion corresponds to the mechanism used by the virus to spread from one cell to others...": Forterre P., "Defining life: the virus viewpoint," *Orig Life Evol Biosph*, 3 Mar 2010: https://www.ncbi.nlm.nih.gov/pmc/articles/PMC2837877/

244 Beijerinck, M., "Ueber ein contagium vivum fluidum als Ursache der Fleckenkrankheit der Tabaksblatter. Verh. Kon. Akad. Wetensch", 1898: https://www.apsnet.org/edcenter/apsnetfeatures/Documents/1998/BeijerckSpotDiseaseTobaccoLeaves.PDF

to a form of sub-microscopic infectious agent that was soluble but unable to be visualized by the technology of the time. In the body of his 1898 paper Beijerinck used the term 'contagium' interchangeably with 'virus'. Although the *Archives of Virology* credits him with the first use of the word virus to mean a new class of pathogen, it is also acknowledged that Beijerinck and his contemporaries would not have envisaged the virus model as it is known today:

> *Beijerinck's claim of a "fluidity" of the contagium is a matter of semantics since he already used it interchangeably with "solubility". His coining of the term "virus" for a new class of pathogens further marks the beginning of a new era in biology. Hence, it is not very fertile to debate the issue who was first in discovering a virus. None of the pioneers could have known what he was talking about.*[245]

It is more than evident that the enigma of what is being talked about extends well beyond the so-called pioneers of virology and continues into the present day. Virology is a unique "science" within the field of biology because of the virologists' propensity to redefine the supposed material nature of the entities they claim to be studying. Changing definitions and the use of linguistic legerdemain can make it difficult for the public to know what they are talking about, if not for the virologists themselves as the following examples illustrate:

> *"My ambition is to show that the word virus has a meaning, and I shall defend a paradoxical viewpoint, namely that viruses are viruses."*
>
> —André Lwoff, 1957[246]

---

[245] Bos, L., "The embryonic beginning of virology: unbiased thinking and dogmatic stagnation," *Archives of Virology*, Jan 1995: https://link.springer.com/content/pdf/10.1007/BF01718437.pdf

[246] Lwoff, A., "The Concept of Virus," *Journal of General Microbiology*, 1957: https://doi.org/10.1099/00221287-17-2-239

> *"...a virus is what virologists say it is...It can be said that virologists invent (and continually reinvent) the concept of a virus as part of the normal progress of their science."*
>
> —William Summers, 2014[247]

> *"Many host districts of the human body and its mucous membranes are heavily 'colonized' by viruses that are not associated with any disease."*
>
> —Editorial, *Clinical Microbiology and Infection*, 2019[248]

> *"...a* [corona]*virus is just a piece of RNA molecule."*
>
> —William Rawlinson, 2020[249]

Whatever the virologists say or consider "normal progress", it is clear that they did not discover viruses in nature and then set about their study of them. The created paradigm is steeped in anti-scientific practices due to its typically unfalsifiable nature - the virologists do not perform experiments in an attempt to falsify their hypothesis because the material existence of viruses has always been assumed in advance. Apparently all that remains is for them to fill in the details:

> *"To the nineteenth-century microbiologist, "virus" was a useful but imprecise concept, defined in operational rather than physical terms. Viruses were thought of in terms of what they do (cause disease, produce lesions on tobacco leaves, and the like), not in terms of what they are."*
>
> —William Summers, 2014[250]

---

247 Summers, W., "Inventing Viruses," *Annual Review of Virology*, Sep 2014: https://doi.org/10.1146/annurev-virology-031413-085432

248 Antonelli, G., Pistello, M., "Virology: a scientific discipline facing new challenges," *Clinical Microbiology and Infection*, 20 Dec 2018: https://doi.org/10.1016/j.cmi.2018.12.003

249 "Covid testing and tracing," *ABC Radio National*, 22 Jun 2020: https://www.abc.net.au/listen/programs/bigideas/covid-testing-and-tracing/12379684

250 Summers, W., "Inventing Viruses," *Annual Review of Virology*, Sep 2014: https://doi.org/10.1146/annurev-virology-031413-085432

In order for viruses to 'do' they must exist first. And if they exist then they must have a specific biochemical composition and function. Since the 1800s their postulated nature has included the aforementioned 'fluid contagium', chemicals, infectious proteins and sub-cellular entities. It was not until the 1950s that the virologists started settling on the modern definition of virus, meaning a resulting contagious particle consisting of a genome (RNA or DNA) surrounded by an encoded proteinaceous coat:

> *Salvador Luria, having published his groundbreaking text* General Virology *in 1953, wrote to* [André] *Lwoff in 1957 with his revised and admittedly clumsy construction of a virus: "I would today define a virus as 'an element of genetic material capable of assuming a transmissible form by incorporation into a transmission apparatus synthesized under the virus' own control'."*[251]

The question still remains as to when the existence of viruses as physical entities was demonstrated? Goodpasture et al. reported on an alleged breakthrough with the, "cultivation of...viruses in the chorio-allantoic membrane of chick embryos" in 1931.[252] However, there was no evidence of any microbe being cultivated and their claim relied on the appearance of, "a vaccinal **lesion** [that] develops and spreads on the membrane." [emphasis added] Here they simply made the assumption that the appearance of a lesion, or damaged membrane tissue, must have been caused by a virus that was present in their introduced sample. A footnote in the paper states that their sample was, "a strain of Levaditi neurovaccine [virus]...kindly supplied by Dr. T. M. Rivers."

Dr Thomas Rivers similarly asserted in advance that his supplied samples contained this "virus" and in his 1930 publication declared it to be a,

---

[251] Ibid.

[252] Goodpasture, E. et al., "The cultivation of vaccine and other viruses in the chorio-allantoic membrane of chick embryos," *Science*, 1931: https://pubmed.ncbi.nlm.nih.gov/17810781/

"Levaditi neurovaccine virus that had been propagated for 6 months in rabbit testicles".[253] It is clear that in all of these experiments the samples were mixed biological specimens and no specific independent variable had been identified. Neither Goodpasture nor Rivers could have possibly known the composition of the so-called 'Levaditi strain'. The tissue in question was evidently diseased and if it caused other exposed tissue to exhibit signs of disease then the nature of the "virus" could not be said to be more than the original meaning of 'poison'.[*254]

It may be argued that this is an unfair charge against these early virologists as their experiments predated the availability of the electron microscope in the late 1930s. However the new nanoscale imaging technology did not help their case as former virologist Dr Stefan Lanka has explained:

> *...the pre-1951 theory of what a virus is supposed to be was refuted by the fact that no one could ever find or photograph anything different in people or animals supposedly infected with a virus from what can be found or photographed in healthy subjects, using the electron microscope. This is still the case today.*[255, *256]

In the 1940s and 1950s, the virologists started favoring the indirect cell culture technique in which specimens from diseased organisms were

---

253 Li C., Rivers, T., "Cultivation of Vaccine Virus," *The Journal of experimental medicine*, 1930: https://doi.org/10.1084/jem.52.4.465

254 *Another example involving misinterpretation of laboratory observations led to the claim of a "Rous Sarcoma Virus" in 1911. In that case there was no evidence of a "virus" in a microbial sense, only noxious substances that caused disease when injected into chickens - see: (p16) Bailey, M., *A Farewell to Virology (Expert Edition)*, 15 Sep 2022: https://drsambailey.com/a-farewell-to-virology-expert-edition/

255 Lanka, S., "Die Verursacher der Corona-Krise sind eindeutig identifiziert Virologen," *wissenschafftplus*, Apr 2020: https://wissenschafftplus.de/uploads/article/wissenschafftplus-virologen.pdf

256 *Claims such as, "viral particles have been demonstrated by electron microscopy in lymph nodes from patients with acquired immune deficiency syndrome," have not been substantiated...(continued on next page)

added to typically abnormal cell lines in the laboratory. If the cells broke down under the microscope, it was then declared that viruses were the cause. However, the cells can also be shown to break down without the addition of any specimen, that is, the procedure itself can cause the same effects.[257] Furthermore, as the present author argued in *Virology's Event Horizon*, there are foundational logical flaws in the cell culture technique:

> *(a) The particles being declared as "viral" are seen for the first time as part of the CPE* [cytopathic effect] *observations, i.e. they are dependent variables. It is preposterous to claim that they are also the independent variable in the same experiment.*
>
> *(b) The in vitro (laboratory) observations cannot be known to replicate an in vivo (within living) process.*
>
> *(c) The techniques involved in electron microscopy introduce further variables that are not controlled, in addition to technical artefact and the further limitation that they are static structures embedded in resin, not living tissue.*[258]

---

256 (cont'd) *For example, in 1988 O'hara et al. examined lymph nodes under electron microscopy and reported that, "in this study, we examined 20 PGL [persistent generalized lymphadenopathy] lymph nodes and found viral particles in 18 cases...In addition we found viral particles, morphologically indistinguishable from those observed in PGL lymph nodes, in 13 of 15 non-HIV related reactive lymph nodes...Clearly, techniques that demonstrate the presence of specific viral antigens or viral RNA are needed to supplement ultrastructural observations": O'Hara C., et al., "The ultrastructural and immunohisto-chemical demonstration of viral particles in lymph nodes from human immunodeficiency virus-related and non-human immunodeficiency virus-related lymphadenopathy syndromes," *Hum Pathol*, May 1988: https://pubmed.ncbi.nlm.nih.gov/3371979/
Their reliance on specific "viral" antigens or RNA requires the demonstration of a virus (in this case an 'HIV' particle) first - something that has not been done - see: Papadopulos-Eleopulos, E., et al., *HIV – A virus like no other*, 12 Jul 2017: www.theperthgroup.com/HIV/TPGVirusLikeNoOther.pdf

257 Bailey, M., *A Farewell to Virology (Expert Edition)*, 15 Sep 2022: https://drsambailey.com/a-farewell-to-virology-expert-edition/

258 Bailey, M., *Virology's Event Horizon*, drsambailey.com, 4 Apr 2024: https://drsambailey.com/virologys-event-horizon/

Like all of the previous experimental methodologies in virology, the cell culture technique did not demonstrate the existence of viruses. It only served to perpetuate a reification fallacy; that is, the *imagined* concept had been inappropriately declared to have a confirmed physical existence.[259] Despite the absence of the requisite evidence, the intangible original formulations of 'virus' from earlier eras was henceforth proclaimed to be a discrete particle possessing parasitic abilities.

The technique of electron microscopy has its own limitations with regard to whether the obtained images can inform us about living cellular biology. Even so, within these limitations the technique should have spelt another dead end for the virus model. It was never able to deliver the anticipated decisive evidence being sought in direct specimens (such as sputum and blood) from people said to have viral illnesses (see again note 256). It was only the cell culture technique that allowed the proliferation of images in biology text books purporting to depict viruses. However, by its very nature, the methodology cannot be controlled for an independent variable and it is impermissible to invent one *post hoc* based on the cell breakdown appearances. Thus, there is no evidence that any of the imaged vesicular structures are pathogenic and contagious entities of exogenous origin.

The virologists employ the 'point and declare' technique in these electron microscopy images such as the example provided in figure 1: the particles are claimed to be SARS-CoV-2 virions and yet there is no corroboration that they are infectious or disease causing. A hypothetical genome is assembled but as the imaged particles were not purified, the provenance of the genetic sequences remains unknown - they could have come from other constituents in the mixture. However, even if they were purified and their biochemical elements determined, that would not automatically qualify them as viruses: the isolated particles would need to be shown to be capable of the required properties as an independent variable in

[259] Ibid.

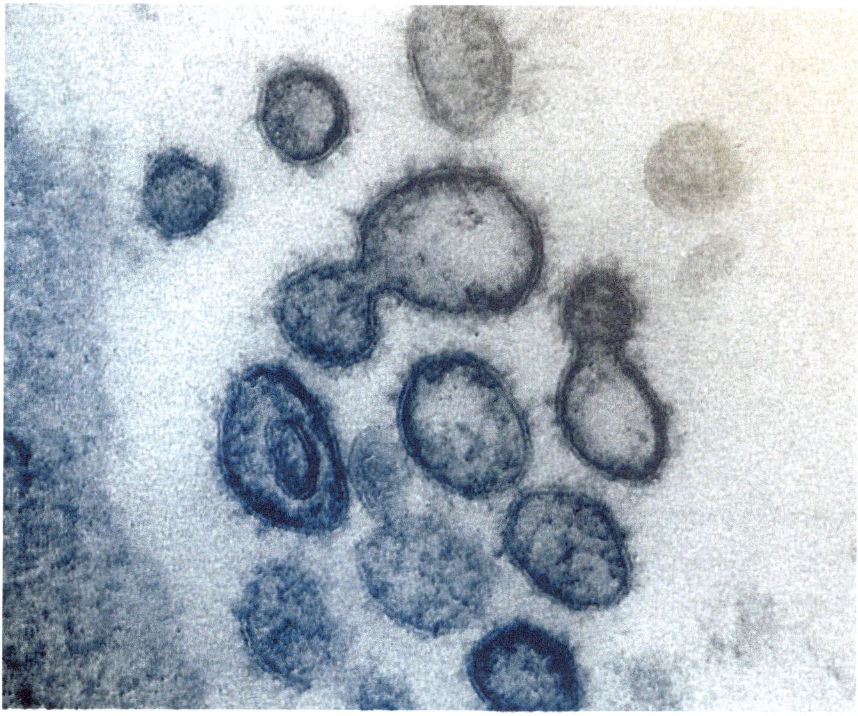

Figure 1. An enhanced electron microscope image made available by the U.S. National Institutes of Health in February 2020. It purports to show 'SARS-CoV-2' virions. No evidence was provided as to how the biological nature or composition of these apparent vesicles was determined. Source: https://www.chicagotribune.com/2020/04/04/know-that-coronavirus-image-with-red-spikes-heres-how-the-artists-at-the-cdc-created-it/

controlled experiments.*[260] The claim that genomics proves the existence of viruses falls back into the same logical fallacy involving the assertion that the viruses are already known to exist in advance. Within virology this applies to both cell cultures and metagenomics (for example, sequencing of clinical samples): there cannot be any "viral" sequences unless viruses are first shown to exist.

260 *Although as outlined in *Virology's Event Horizon*, an over-riding problem remains: these particles are observations in a cell culture experiment, not independent variables found directly in nature.

The central tenet of the virus model is mired in a fallacy of circular reasoning that its proponents appear unwilling to address. In 2014, it was stated in the *Annual Review of Virology* that:

> *The **basic idea** that viruses are the material basis for disease transmission has changed little in the past 150 years; what has changed is our understanding of the essential properties and biological capacities of viruses...The concept of a virus has particularly been determined by technological advances rather than scientific understanding.*[261] [emphasis added]

However, this "basic idea" has never been established and, in accordance with the scientific method, the concept of 'virus' remains as it was in the 1800s: a mental construct that attempts to explain why organisms become diseased. Without a tangible independent variable, no other indirect observations or technological developments can rescue the model from this fatal gap in the evidence.

Bacteriophage

Bacteriophage literally means bacteria devourer or eater.[262] The term was coined by Félix d'Hérelle in 1917 when he declared, "I have isolated an invisible microbe endowed with an antagonistic property against the bacillus of Shiga [*Shigella dysenteriae*]."[263] It was a nonsensical, if not paradoxical statement as he did not demonstrate the physical isolation of anything. The "invisible microbe" once again invoked a reification fallacy where he attempted to materialize a mental construct through a linguistic sleight of hand. Nevertheless, the story was embraced by the virology

261 Summers, W., "Inventing Viruses," *Annual Review of Virology*, Sep 2014: https://doi.org/10.1146/annurev-virology-031413-085432

262 https://www.etymonline.com/word/bacteriophage#etymonline_v_26860

263 d'Hérelle, F., "Sur un microbe invisible antagoniste des bacilles dysentériques" [An invisible microbe that is antagonistic to the dysentery bacillus], *Comptes rendus Acad. Sciences*, 1917: https://web.archive.org/web/20110511183504/http://202.114.65.51/fzjx/wsw/wswfzjs/pdf/1917p157.pdf

establishment and in the 2010 edition of the *Desk Encyclopedia of General Virology* we are told, "d'Hérelle understood immediately that he had found a new category of viruses".[264]

D'Hérelle's "anti-Shiga microbe" was created by adding four or five drops of feces to a broth, incubating the mixture at 37°C for 18 hours and then passing the contents through a Chamberland candle filter (to remove bacterial cells).[265] He observed that the addition of this cell-free filtrate to a culture of Shigella bacteria inhibited their growth and resulted in their lysis. In line with other virologists he had simply invented a hypothetical entity, the bacteriophage, to explain the cause of an observation in the bacterial culture. Rather than being skeptical of his own guesswork about a parasitic "invisible microbe" in his mixture he continued to make all subsequent observations fit his unestablished premise:

> *The antagonistic microbe can never be cultivated in media in the absence of the dysentery bacillus. It does not attack heat-killed dysentery bacilli, but is cultivated perfectly in a suspension of washed cells in physiological saline.*[266]

Authors in the modern era have continued to promulgate the claims of d'Hérelle as if they were unquestionable scientific facts. Some of them have made their own additions to the story, even going so far as to award teleological properties to the imagined bacterial "viruses":

> [D'Hérelle] *quickly learned that bacteriophages are found wherever bacteria thrive: in sewers, in rivers that catch waste runoff from pipes, and in the stool of convalescent patients.*

---

[264] Ackermann, H., "History of Virology: Bacteriophages" in *Desk Encyclopedia of General Virology*, Elsevier, 2010: https://books.google.com.au/books

[265] d'Hérelle, F., "Sur un microbe invisible antagoniste des bacilles dysentériques" [An invisible microbe that is antagonistic to the dysentery bacillus], *Comptes rendus Acad. Sciences*, 1917: https://web.archive.org/web/20110511183504/http://202.114.65.51/fzjx/wsw/wswfzjs/pdf/1917p157.pdf

[266] Ibid.

> *Like any predator, bacteriophages are best able to survive and multiply when they are in close proximity to their food supply, where they fulfil their evolutionary role of keeping bacteria in check.*[267]

The first electron micrographs showing purported bacteriophages were published in 1940 in two papers from Germany and according to the journal *Bacteriophage*, "proved the particulate nature of bacteriophages."[268] One paper described the imaging of a mixture made by, "adding a lysate to a broth culture of *E. coli*".[269] Two images from the paper can be seen in figure 2. The vesicular particles around the cells were declared to be viral in nature presumably as this had already been decided in advance. The possibility that the particles were originally endogenous and a result of the breakdown of the cells was not apparently considered by the authors in their conclusions.

The other 1940 publication reported on electron microscopy of a "filtered bacteria-free phage lysate of a broth culture of coli bacteria".[270] This imaging provided some evidence of homogeneous particles around 60 nanometers in diameter - however, like the first paper there was no demonstration that these were viral in nature.

There are many known precipitants of cell membrane lysis including pressure, heating, osmotic shock, alkali exposure, detergents, and

---

267 Kuchment, A., "Helpful Little Bodies" in *The Forgotten Cure - The Past and Future of Phage Therapy*, Springer, 2012: https://link.springer.com/book/10.1007/978-1-4614-0251-0

268 Ackermann, H., "The first phage electron micrographs," *Bacteriophage*, 1 Jul 2011: https://doi.org/10.4161%2Fbact.1.4.17280

269 Ruska, H., "Visualization of bacteriophage lysis in the hypermicroscope," *Naturwissenschaften*, 1940: https://www.ncbi.nlm.nih.gov/pmc/articles/PMC3626388/ (German and English)

270 Pfankuch, E., Kausche, G., "Isolation and supra-microscopic representation of a bacteriophage," *Naturwissenschaften*, 1940: https://www.ncbi.nlm.nih.gov/pmc/articles/PMC3626389/ (German and English)

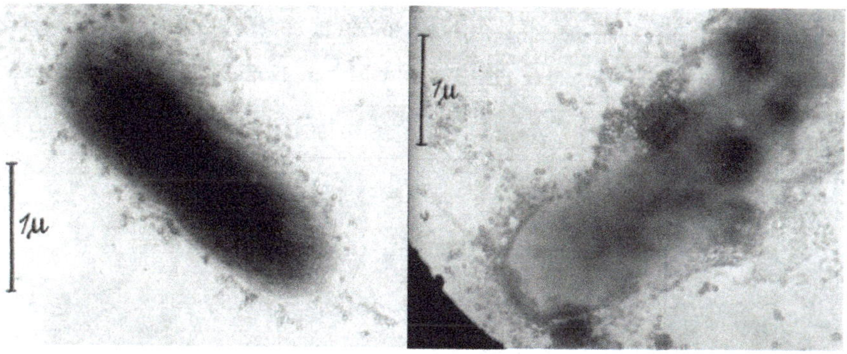

Figure 2. Some of the first published electron micrographs in 1940 of "coliphages" imagined to be "attacking" the surface of an *Escherichia coli* bacterium. Source: https://www.ncbi.nlm.nih.gov/pmc/articles/PMC3626388/figure/F1/

enzymes as well as sonic, optical and electrical insults.[271] Figure 3 below shows the breakdown of *Escherichia coli* cells following exposure to pVEC, a disrupting peptide that is 18 amino acids in length. Note that the particles surrounding the cells were not called 'bacteriophages' in this instance.

In 2015, Dr Stefan Lanka outlined why the virologists' preconceived idea about predatory bacterial "viruses" led them to the wrong conclusions when interpreting the images:

> *Due to the belief that these - at the time of their discovery still invisible - structures were killing the bacteria, they were called phages/bacteriophages, "eaters of bacteria". Only later it was determined that merely highly inbred and therefore almost non-viable bacteria can be made to turn into phages, or bacteria which are being destroyed so fast that they do not have time to form spores.*[272]

---

271 Shehadul Islam, M. et al., "A Review on Macroscale and Microscale Cell Lysis Methods," *Micromachines (Basel)*, 8 Mar 2017: https://doi.org/10.3390%2Fmi8030083

272 Lanka, S., "Dismantling the Virus Theory," *wissenschafftplus*, Jun 2015: http://dx.doi.org/10.13140/RG.2.2.29743.33447

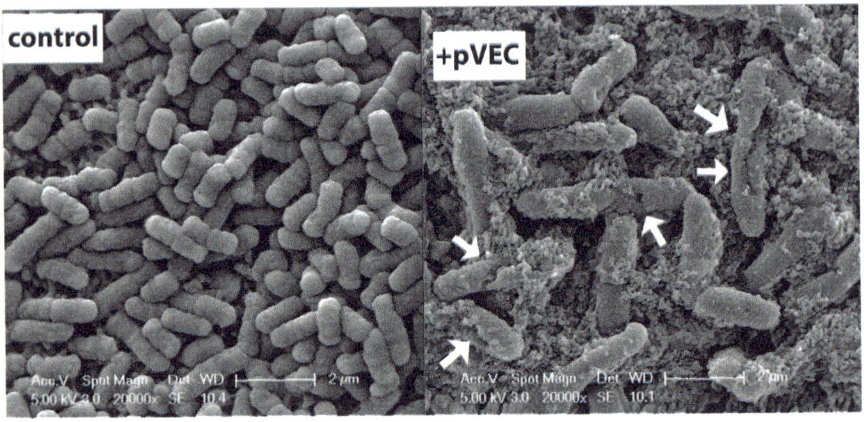

Figure 3. Scanning electron micrographs showing the lysis of *E.coli* cells after exposure to pVEC, an 18 amino acid long cell-penetrating peptide. Source: https://www.mdpi.com/2218-273X/8/3/77

Bacteriophages exist in so far as they can be found in nature, isolated and characterized. They can and will be found everywhere that bacteria are found. In the ocean, they may be seen in quantities of up to 10^8/milliliter of water and thousands have been described in phage databases.[273] The fault lies in the name - they are not "bacteria eating" particles and can only be said to be endogenous elements that are part of a reaction to environmental changes in microbiological systems.

The virologists have never been able to show the existence of pathogenic viruses and have compounded their errors by first claiming that bacteriophages are viral in nature and then implying that there are equivalent viral particles that attack larger organisms such as humans.*[274]

273 https://phagescope.deepomics.org/database/phage

274 *Even if 'bacteriophages' were shown to be parasitic it would still not be evidence for pathogenic viruses in humans and other multicellular organisms.

Single "Virus" Genomics

Flow cytometry is a technique that allows for the analysis of single biological cells by passing a fluid sample through a narrow sheath. A laser beam is directed at the sheath and detectors receive optical and impedance signals that provide information about the cells as they flow past.[275] Some flow cytometry instruments can also be used to physically separate particular cell types. It is a tool that has been used for decades in medical diagnostics and scientific research.

By the 1980s, flow cytometry was being used to quantify microscopic phytoplankton in natural water samples.[276] In the 1990s it was claimed that, "flow cytometry (FCM) was successfully used to enumerate viruses in seawater".[277] However, the "viruses" that were measured were of the *Phaeocystis* class, a "virioplankton" or bacteriophage related to phytoplankton. Once again and without substantive evidence, the virologists have declared that they are viral in nature with bacteriophages being described as being part of an "infection" cycle rather than a microbial *life* cycle. Review papers such as one published in 2000 continue to note that wherever microbes are active, so too are their bacteriophages:

> *For aquatic viruses, abundance has, in nearly every case that has been examined, correlated most strongly with bacterioplankton concentration. Furthermore, it appears that larger virioplankton populations are found under conditions of high bacterial productivity. Many authors have speculated*

---

[275] "Flow cytometry," *Wikipedia*: https://en.wikipedia.org/wiki/Flow_cytometry (accessed 7 Jul 2024)

[276] Olson, R. et al., "Marine phytoplankton distributions measured using shipboard flow cytometry," *Deep Sea Research Part A. Oceanographic Research Papers*, Oct 1985: https://www.sciencedirect.com/science/article/abs/pii/0198014985900093

[277] Marie, D. et al., "Enumeration of marine viruses in culture and natural samples by flow cytometry," *Appl Environ Microbiol*, Jan 1999: https://www.ncbi.nlm.nih.gov/pmc/articles/PMC90981/#B20

> *that bacteriophages comprise the majority of virioplankton populations. Thus, it is not surprising that the abundance of aquatic viruses is closely correlated with the abundance and activity of bacterioplankton.*[278]

As Dr Stefan Lanka has explained, the existence of bacteriophages and giant viruses as well-defined physical particles found in nature is not being questioned. However, the names of these two related entities are misnomers and their biological role has not been shown to be one of parasitism:

> *...the so-called giant viruses, i.e. an enwrapped nucleic acid that can be found everywhere in the sea and in basic organisms. Like all bacterial phages, not only they are harmless, but they have beneficial functions. They can be also isolated by using the density gradient centrifugation, which proves their existence.*[279]

While these biological paradigms are ignored, further developments in flow cytometry led to the announcement of "single virus genomics" (SVG) in a 2011 *Public Library of Science* publication.[280] It was claimed that, "the benefits of SVG will be far-reaching, enabling novel virus discovery in a variety of clinical and environmental settings..."[281] The technique apparently isolated single particles into agarose droplets which was confirmed by Confocal Laser Scanning Microscopy. The isolated particles were then DNA sequenced through genomic amplification. An incredible

---

[278] Wommack K. & Colwell R., "Virioplankton: viruses in aquatic ecosystems," *Microbiol Mol Biol Rev*, Mar 2000: https://www.ncbi.nlm.nih.gov/pmc/articles/PMC98987/

[279] Lanka, S., "Dismantling the Virus Theory," *wissenschafftplus*, Jun 2015: http://dx.doi.org/10.13140/RG.2.2.29743.33447

[280] Allen L. et al., "Single virus genomics: a new tool for virus discovery," *PLoS One*, 23 Mar 2011: https://www.ncbi.nlm.nih.gov/pmc/articles/PMC3059205/

[281] Ibid.

triumph of technology this may be but the paper did not actually demonstrate that these particles were viruses. The tested "viral" suspensions were *E. coli* T4 and lambda bacteriophages - the nature of which have been already discussed in the present paper.

SVG cannot enable "virus discovery" unless it can first be shown that viruses, as pathological microbial entities, exist. The tautological declaration that, "a virus is what virologists say it is," is illustrative of a scientifically bankrupt paradigm. Humanity has been led to believe the virologists are studying microbes that are both contagious and disease-causing. There has been a bombardment of information concerning genomics, proteomics, electron micrographs, alleged diagnostic tests and epidemiological data. The virologists may believe that such data continues to fit the model first conceived in the 19th century but these imaginings have no bearing on biological reality.

ACKNOWLEDGEMENTS

In no particular order the following individuals have influenced my writing on the subject of virology: Dr Valendar Turner, Eleni Papadopulos-Eleopulos, Mike Stone, Torsten Engelbrecht, Dr Claus Köhnlein, Dr Andrew Kaufman, Dr Thomas Cowan, Dr Samantha Bailey, David Crowe, Dr Stefan Lanka, Dr John Bevan-Smith, Dr Kary Mullis, Christine Massey, Dr Ulric Williams, Daniel Roytas.

ABOUT THE AUTHOR

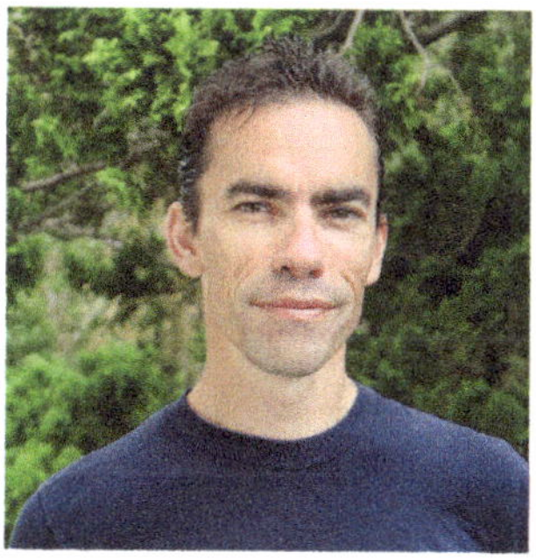

Dr Mark Bailey, MB ChB, PGDipMSM, MHealSc is a microbiology, medical industry and health researcher who worked in medical practice, including clinical trials, for two decades. With his wife, Dr Sam Bailey, the couple have made their extensive collection of medical and health information freely available through their website drsambailey.com.

Made in the USA
Monee, IL
30 October 2026

67079974R00075